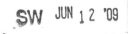

10u Question About How to Quit Smoking

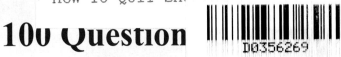

D0356269

Charles Herrick, MD

Department of Psychiatry
Danbury Hospital
Danbury, CT
New York Medical College
Valhalla, NY

Charlotte Herrick, PhD, RN

Professor Emeritas
School of Nursing
University of North Carolina
Greensboro, NC

Marianne Mitchell, APRN

Pulmonary Department
Danbury Hospital
Danbury, CT

JONES AND BARTLETT PUBLISHERS
Sudbury, Massachusetts
BOSTON   TORONTO   LONDON   SINGAPORE

World Headquarters

Jones and Bartlett Publishers
40 Tall Pine Drive
Sudbury, MA 01776
978-443-5000
info@jbpub.com
www.jbpub.com

Jones and Bartlett Publishers
Canada
6339 Ormindale Way
Mississauga, Ontario L5V 1J2
Canada

Jones and Bartlett Publishers
International
Barb House, Barb Mews
London W6 7PA
United Kingdom

Jones and Bartlett's books and products are available through most bookstores and online booksellers. To contact Jones and Bartlett Publishers directly, call 800-832-0034, fax 978-443-8000, or visit our website, www.jbpub.com.

Substantial discounts on bulk quantities of Jones and Bartlett's publications are available to corporations, professional associations, and other qualified organizations. For details and specific discount information, contact the special sales department at Jones and Bartlett via the above contact information or send an email to specialsales@jbpub.com.

The authors, editor, and publisher have made every effort to provide accurate information. However, they are not responsible for errors, omissions, or for any outcomes related to the use of the contents of this book and take no responsibility for the use of the products and procedures described. Treatments and side effects described in this book may not be applicable to all people; likewise, some people may require a dose or experience a side effect that is not described herein. Drugs and medical devices are discussed that may have limited availability controlled by the Food and Drug Administration (FDA) for use only in a research study or clinical trial. Research, clinical practice, and government regulations often change the accepted standard in this field. When consideration is being given to use of any drug in the clinical setting, the health care provider or reader is responsible for determining FDA status of the drug, reading the package insert, and reviewing prescribing information for the most up-to-date recommendations on dose, precautions, and contraindications, and determining the appropriate usage for the product. This is especially important in the case of drugs that are new or seldom used.

Production Credits
Publisher: Christopher Davis
Senior Editorial Assistant: Jessica Acox
Associate Production Editor: Leah Corrigan
Marketing Manager: Ilana Goddess
V.P., Manufacturing and Inventory Control:
   Therese Connell
Composition: Lynn L'Heureux

Cover Design: Carolyn Downer
Cover Images: © Zdenka Micka/ShutterStock, Inc.
   © Anita/ShutterStock, Inc.
   © Christy Thompson/ShutterStock, Inc.
   © Patrick Sheandell O'Carroll/PhotoAlto/
   PictureQuest
Printing and Binding: Malloy, Inc.
Cover Printing: Malloy, Inc.

Library of Congress Cataloging-in-Publication Data
Herrick, Charles.
  100 questions & answers about how to quit smoking / Charles Herrick, Charlotte Herrick, Marianne Mitchell.
     p. cm.
  Includes index.
  ISBN 978-0-7637-5741-0 (alk. paper)
  1. Smoking. 2. Smoking cessation. I. Herrick, Charlotte A. (Charlotte Anne), 1933- II. Mitchell, Marianne. III. Title. IV. Title: One hundred questions and answers about how to quit smoking.
  HV5740.H47 2009
  616.86'5--dc22

6048   2008047289

Printed in the United States of America
13 12 11 10 09   10 9 8 7 6 5 4 3 2 1

To my wife, Ana Cristina, whose involved critical reading, frequent meetings with the co-authors, and editorial efforts justly deserve the right to be considered as a co-author to this book as well. It would not have been written and completed without her organizing force.

—Charles Herrick, MD

This book is dedicated to my husband, children, and grandchildren. I am a proud wife, mother, and grandmother.

I want to thank my son, Charles Herrick, for inviting me to co-author a second book with him. I am also grateful to his wife for the support that she provided both of us in bringing this book to fruition. Her editorial contributions were invaluable.

I especially want to thank my husband, Bob Herrick, for his patience in allowing me the time to do the research and writing that contributed to making *100 Questions & Answers about How to Quit Smoking* possible. He has continued to encourage me to write and over the past few years I have written three books, all published by Jones and Bartlett. I want to thank the editorial staff of Jones and Bartlett. It has been gratifying to work with all of you.

I would also like to dedicate this book to all of the smokers who have quit smoking. Congratulations! As an ex-smoker, I know how hard it was. This dedication also includes those smokers who are valiantly trying to quit. Keep trying and eventually you will succeed! I am deeply grateful to two friends and colleagues who read parts of this book and gave suggestions. One is an ex-smoker, who shared her journey with me, and the other is currently trying to quit, using the patch. The fact that she is trying to stop smoking after reading parts of this book is a testament to the fact that *100 Questions & Answers about How to Quit Smoking* may be helpful. Thank you so much. I hope both of you live healthy and productive lives.

—Charlotte A. Herrick, PhD, RN

I dedicate this book to my husband, Scott, and my kids, Megan, Jillian, and Drew. They have put up with my smoking cessation ramblings for many years and can probably recite the dangers of smoking in their sleep. I could not have done this without you.

—Marianne Mitchell, APRN

Tobacco has probably had a bigger impact on the lives of Americans than all plants, drugs, or other commodities combined. This may sound exaggerated, but when one examines the history of our nation one cannot but be left with the feeling that, were it not for tobacco, we would not have been able to gain our independence as rapidly as we did. Tobacco did it all. It brought jobs and opportunity. It led to rapid agricultural development. It brought wealth, and with wealth came the power to obtain independence. Unfortunately, like all things that seem initially like windfalls, the cultivation of tobacco came at a price. That price was paid, in many respects, on the backs of African Americans, who worked the plantations to bring the plant to market and fuel the American economy. (Cotton contributed to this as well, but tobacco was the first cash crop.) Gradually, however, America's increasing dependency on slave labor for that cash crop created deep divisions, which finally ignited in the form of a bloody Civil War, the effects of which are still being felt today over a hundred years later.

In a sense, tobacco's story on the social level has mirrored its effects on the individual level. Unlike any other drug of its kind, tobacco does it all. It perks you up and makes you sharper, but it also slows you down and allows you to focus better so you can block out bothersome stimuli; It stimulates and it sedates. It helps you manage everything that stress can throw your way without impairing you or turning you into an idiot. Because of this wealth of activity, of providing for every psychological need in a steady and manageable way, tobacco creates a slow but certain dependency that catches you off-guard until a civil war erupts in your body in the form of some life threatening disease that you can conveniently ignore until it explodes, leaving you at the edge of health.

We now approach smokers in the same way we approached other social outcasts, looking at them with disdain, viewing them as moral failures at best, or hooligans at worst. We wonder how they can ignore the flood of information that drowns us all with horrific statistics about rates of cancer and heart disease and emphysema, all leading to lost years and lost quality of life. We forget our past. We forget that this attitude is the exception, not the rule. We forget that even if we never smoked, our parents smoked, and smoking was part of the fabric of our lives, invading every medium as surely as the smoke filled restaurants, airplanes, bars, and homes filled our lungs as an accepted part of life. Smoking was the engine of America's success in the eighteenth and nineteenth centuries, just as oil has been America's success in the twentieth. While one can hope for a future of independence from both, one cannot forget to pay proper respect to the fact that our current freedoms and standard of living have been partly built on these products.

It is an unfortunate fact of human nature to make things all good or all bad. It is especially unfortunate that Americans tend to do this more than other peoples. It is unfortunate because it often leads us to act in ways that ultimately hurt us rather than help us. While it is a good thing that we have become more aware of the dangers of second hand smoke and have created laws to limit our exposure to it, it is not a good thing to treat our family and friends who smoke as pariahs. Hopefully, this book will provide some insight and understanding regarding tobacco's insidious effects on our biology, while offering hope that effective treatment is available to enable us to ultimately free ourselves from its grasp.

PART ONE

The Basics

What is tobacco?

How do chemicals such as nicotine work
in the brain?

What are the psychological effects of nicotine?

More...

1. What is tobacco?

Tobacco is a plant that was domesticated, cultivated, and used by Native Americans for at least the past 5000 years, long before Columbus arrived in America. It is believed that the plant originated from South America and its cultivation spread northward during prehistoric times. Tobacco may even be the first domesticated plant in the Americas, as it was more widely cultivated by Native Americans than maize at the time the first Europeans arrived. Tobacco is the fastest spreading plant in human history. From the Americas, the Spanish conquistadors and early European explorers carried it to Europe where its cultivation rapidly spread to Asia.

Tobacco is the fastest spreading plant in human history.

Numerous species are native to South America, Mexico, and the West Indies. The plant grows 4 to 6 feet high and bears pink flowers. It has huge leaves. The tobacco plant, *Nicotiana tabacum*, was named after Jean Nicot, the French ambassador to Portugal who first brought the plant back from Brazil in 1560. A number of tobacco species grow naturally in the Americas, all belonging to the genus *Nicotiana* of the *Solanacease* family. Products manufactured from the leaf are used in cigars, cigarettes, snuff, pipes, and chewing tobacco. The chief commercial species is *N. tabacum*, which is native to tropical America. *N. rustica* was grown in Virginia and the Carolinas during the Colonial era. Although today the number of tobacco farms is declining, it remains the chief crop in the Mid-Atlantic, Southeastern states, and some of the Southern states, including Kentucky and Tennessee. Many American farmers have exchanged their tobacco crops for other products. Today, vineyards are developing all over North Carolina to replace the old tobacco farms. *N. rustica* is also grown in Turkey, Russia, and other parts of the Ottoman Empire, and is known as Turkish Tobacco.

Tobacco requires a warm climate and rich, well-drained soil. The leaves are picked as they mature and are harvested together with the stalk. After harvesting, the tobacco leaves are cured, fermented, and aged to develop an aroma and to reduce the harsh taste. There are several methods of curing tobacco leaves. Fire curing involves drying the leaves in smoke. Air curing involves hanging the leaves to dry in a well-ventilated structure. Another form of curing is when the leaves are dried by radiant heat from flues or pipes connected to a furnace.

Once the leaves are cured, the tobacco leaves are graded, bunched, and stacked into piles, and then put in closed containers for fermentation and aging. Most commercial tobacco is a blend of different types of tobacco. Other ingredients such as maple sugar and other sugars are then added for taste.

2. Why do people use tobacco?

Tobacco is clearly valued for its **psychoactive** effects. This means that it has several actions on the mind that depend upon the dose used. It can be used to stimulate the mind, relieve anxiety, or create visions or hallucinations. All of these properties can be pleasurable. In many Native American tribes, tobacco was traditionally used for religious or shamanistic purposes. Traditionally, tobacco was reserved primarily for shamans and priests because of its hallucinogenic properties. Tobacco was thought to allow the individual a conduit to the visions of the future, to the afterlife, God, or to a greater spiritual plain. All parts of the plant were used for different medicinal purposes; tobacco was used in agriculture to deter insects and other plant diseases, and it was a source of currency (see Question 4). Many tribes use tobacco to this day in their ceremonies and consider it one of the most important of their sacred herbs.

During the Colonial era, tobacco was used as a commodity for bartering, and it was exported to Europe in exchange for manufactured products. Snuff and chewing tobacco were initially more popular among men before the Civil War. Starting with World War I, cigarettes became popular among Americans (see Question 3). Snuff, chewing tobacco, cigars, pipes, and cigarettes are all used for pleasure. Nicotine, the major psychoactive ingredient of tobacco, can act as both a stimulant to enhancing the ability to think clearly and improve

Psychoactive

A drug or chemical substance that acts on the brain to alter mood, behavior, perception, or consciousness. Abuse of some of these substances may cause addiction.

alertness, and as a relaxant to relieve anxiety, so that the smoker "feels good." (Question 83 reviews nicotine's possible health benefits.)

3. What is the history of tobacco use?

The following is a timeline of the history of tobacco.

- Before 1492: Tobacco was first used by the pre-Columbian Americans, who cultivated it for ceremonial and medicinal purposes.

- 1492: Christopher Columbus arrived in the Caribbean and observed the natives smoking and chewing tobacco. The Indians smoked tobacco through a Y shaped pipe called a *Tobago*. Christopher Columbus brought a few tobacco leaves and seeds back to Europe.

- 1556: Tobacco did not gain popularity until it was introduced to France in 1556, when Jean Nicot, a Frenchman, gave the tobacco seeds to Catherine de Medicis, the Queen of France. Plants grew from the seeds and were christened *Nicotine tabacur* after Jean Nicot's name. Later, the addictive substance was called **nicotine**.

Nicotine

A chemical found in a variety of plants that targets a specific group of acetylcholine receptors known as nicotinic receptors.

- 1584: Sir Francis Drake, the famous explorer of California Coast, introduced tobacco to Sir Walter Raleigh, another well-known explorer of the Carolinas.

- 1612: The first commercial tobacco crop was grown in Virginia.

- 1619: The first African slaves were brought to Jamestown, Virginia to work the tobacco plantations. Later in 1661, slavery was officially legalized in Virginia.

- 1730: The first tobacco factories opened up to manufacture snuff.

- 1761: One of the first investigations about the relationship between tobacco and disease concluded that malignancies of the respiratory tract, including the nose, could be traced to the use of snuff.

- 1776: The American Revolution occurred in part because of "A Tobacco War." Colonists objected to the taxes levied on their tobacco products by British merchants. Tobacco also served as collateral during the American Revolution, which helped to finance the French involvement.

- Mid-18th Century: "Big Tobacco" was born including its manufacturers Duke, Philip Morris, Liggett, and J.R. Reynolds. After the inventions of matches and later lighters, the number of cigarette smokers skyrocketed.

- 1861: Tobacco was issued along with food rations and drink to soldiers during the Civil War. Many Northerners were first introduced to tobacco during the Civil War. Hand-rolled cigarettes became popular. Before 1861, tobacco was generally smoked in pipes or cigars.

- 1864: The first cigarette factory was built in the United States.

- 1881: James E. Bonsack invented an automated cigarette making machine, sponsored by the Duke Company, which could produce 200 cigarettes per minute. Prior to this invention, 50 workers were required to produce 200 cigarettes. This invention markedly reduced the costs of production.

- 1906: Tobacco was removed from the *U.S. Pharmacopeia*, thus eliminating The Federal Drug Administration's (FDA) ability to regulate tobacco use.

- 1909: Per capita smoking consumption grew, especially among men, who smoked mostly cigars and pipes.

- 1912: The first lobectomy for lung cancer was performed.

- 1917: During World War I, cigarettes were favored over pipes and cigars because they were more portable during combat. Between 1910 and 1919, the production of cigarettes increased by 633%.

- 1929: Mt. Zion Hospital in San Francisco performed six successful lobectomies. This was the start of modern thoracic surgery.

- 1933: The first successful pneumonectomy was performed for lung cancer.

- 1936: Dr Alan Oschner first saw lung cancer in 1919. Afterward, Oschner saw nine patients with lung cancer within a six month period. He concluded that the cause was cigarette smoking.

- 1945: It became socially acceptable for women to smoke. During World War II, The American Red Cross and other organizations distributed cigarettes to men and women in uniform.

- 1946: The "Golden Age" of advertising began promoting the use of cigarettes to the general public.

- 1954: The "Marlboro Man" ad was introduced by Phillip Morris, to promote the idea that men who smoke are more masculine and virile. The American Medical Association Board banned all advertising of tobacco and alcohol in their publications.

- 1959: The Surgeon General published the U.S. Public Health Services' position that cigarette smoking causes lung cancer.

- 1964: The first *Surgeon General's Report on Smoking and Health* was published. Ten scientists spent 14 months reviewing the scientific literature from all over the world. Per capita consumption dropped by 2% after the publication of the report. This report was pivotal in changing the smoking habits of Americans.

- 1971: Tobacco companies could no longer advertise in the broadcast media, which included television and radio. However, the ban did not include advertising in magazines and newspapers.

- 1986: The 19th *Surgeon General's Report* reported that smokeless tobacco (chewing tobacco and snuff) is addictive.

- 1987: The U.S. Congress banned smoking on airline flights of less than two hours.

- 1992: Wayne McLaren, the world-famous "Marlboro Man," died of lung cancer at the age of 51.

- 1994: Mississippi became the first state to sue tobacco companies for the cost of health care associated with smoking-related diseases. Other states followed. FDA announced it could consider regulating nicotine in cigarettes as a drug in response to a Citizen's Petition by the Coalition on Smoking OR Health.

- 1996: FDA declared cigarettes to be "drug delivery devices." Restrictions were proposed on marketing and sales to reduce the incidence of smoking by young people.

- 1996: Scientists announced that they found a direct chemical link between a substance found in tobacco tar and the development of cancer. Lawsuits proliferated in Minnesota, Mississippi, West Virginia, and Florida for smokers seeking reimbursements from the states for the costs of medical care for smoking-related illnesses.

- 1997: Nonsmoking bars became the norm in California. In San Francisco, the Board of Supervisors, with prodding from the San Francisco Medical Society and other anti-smoking and health-related groups, banned outdoor advertising of tobacco products.

- 1998: Forty-six States' attorney generals and the tobacco industry arrived at a settlement with four of the largest tobacco companies in the United States, known as the Tobacco Master Settlement Agreement (MSA). (More on MSA in Question 95.) The States agreed to limit further lawsuits against the tobacco industry in exchange for higher taxes on cigarettes to pay for the States' tobacco-related medical expenses. Tobacco companies also agreed to compensate the States $206 billion to establish tobacco smoking prevention programs.

- 1999: Phillip Morris admitted publicly that smoking causes cancer.

- 2000: The U.S. Supreme Court, upholding an earlier decision in the Food and Drug Administration v. Brown & Williamson Tobacco Corp. et al., ruled 5 to 4 that the FDA did not have authority to regulate tobacco as a drug. Within weeks of this ruling, FDA revoked its final rule, issued in 1996, that restricted the sale and distribution of cigarettes and smokeless tobacco products to children and adolescents, and that determined that cigarettes and smokeless tobacco products are combination products consisting of a drug (nicotine) and device components intended to deliver nicotine to the body.

- 1950–2004: The proportion of adult smokers in the United States declined from a high of 46% in the 1950s to a low of 21% in 2004.

- 2004–2008: Smoking continues to decline in American society, but because of globalization, its use continues to grow internationally.

4. What are the different ways in which tobacco is consumed?

Tobacco can be ingested in many forms. Native Americans produced tobacco to be consumed as a beverage but mainly ingested it by smoking it using a pipe. A paste of moistened tobacco applied to the skin was a common remedy for insect bites and stings, and tobacco has been used to control minor bleeding as well as an antiseptic, as it kills many bacteria. Occasionally, it was used medicinally as an enema, but this method was far too dangerous because the high risk of overdose. It was therefore limited to smoking by shamans as a method for achieving visions.

Chewing and snorting are also utilized. Finally, tobacco is absorbed easily through the skin, and people have been known to put snuff between their toes as a method of remaining inconspicuous while using it.

Cigarette smoking gained popularity after the Civil War when cigarette sales surged. By the twentieth century, the growth of cigarette smoking was exponential across all classes of people, both males and females.

Pipes

Traditionally, indigenous people of North and South America used pipe ceremonies to celebrate their religious and community festivals. Sacred pipes are still commonly used today as they were in the past for traditional Native American ceremonies. Pipe smoking also occurred at the completion of a bargain or contract. Traditionally, people who belonged to the tribes of North and South America did not use tobacco outside of these highly ritualized occasions. Because tobacco was considered a gift from the Gods, misusing it would result in an illness that was considered to be from the wrath of the Gods or Spirits.

Cigarettes

Today and during most of the twentieth century, cigarette smoking is the most common method of tobacco use. After the Civil War, the shift to cigarette smoking from chewing tobacco, snuff, and pipe smoking, constituted a profound change in the production and consumption of tobacco. The earliest cigarettes were made during the seventeenth century and were wrapped in cornhusks. Following the Civil War, Duke & Company (based in Durham NC) was one of the first companies to mass-produce cigarettes. The tobacco manufacturer also produced other tobacco products. Duke began packaging cigarettes in 1879. Duke is considered the "father" of the modern tobacco industry, which has dominated the American economy from that time until now. As late as the 1920s, it was still unclear which method of tobacco use would be the most popular, but by the late 1930s and 1940s, cigarettes were the most widely manufactured form of tobacco among Americans.

Today and during most of the 20th century, cigarette smoking is the most common method of tobacco use.

The Basics

Cigars

Cigars are not as easily mass-produced as are cigarettes. Manufacturing cigars is more labor intensive, as the tobacco leaves are hand rolled, and therefore cigars are more expensive and not marketed as extensively as other forms of tobacco. Educated urban and well-to-do men enjoyed a pipe or cigar because tobacco smoking was a symbol of power during the late 1800s and the early 1900s. Cigars and pipes were typically smoked in men's parlors and drawing rooms. The transition from cigars and pipes to cigarettes occurred during and after World War I and continued through World War II. By the end of WWII, cigarettes were clearly the most popular means of tobacco use by rich and poor alike. After the Cuban Missile Crisis, Cuban cigars were banned from importation to the United States, which also contributed to an increase in the U.S. cigarette market.

Snuff

In some Native American tribes, tobacco was used by medicine men for its medicinal properties and was frequently chewed. Snuff was popular during the seventeenth and eighteenth centuries throughout the United States and Europe. Snuff is a generic term for fine-ground smokeless tobacco. European snuff is generally snorted while American snuff is generally dipped. Dry snuff is sniffed up the nose. Dipped snuff is a moist tobacco paste that is held between the cheek or lip and the gums, allowing the nicotine to be absorbed in that manner. Until the early twentieth century, snuff dipping was popular in rural America, especially in the South. Popular brands of snuff were Copenhagen, Skoal, Timber Wolf, Chisholm, Grizzly, and Kodiak, and many of these brands are still found in tobacco shops today. Some smokeless tobacco, such as Kodiak, contains a higher dose of nicotine than cigarettes. Snuff can damage human organs and lead to cancer of the mouth and other types of cancers as well as heart disease and other illnesses. Badly stained teeth are found in smokeless tobacco users.

Chewing Tobacco

For many years, chewing tobacco was the most common means of using tobacco. Native Americans in both North and South America chewed the leaves of tobacco, which were frequently mixed with lime. The "twist" is the oldest form of chewing tobacco. Three high quality tobacco leaves are braided together and twisted into a rope and then cured. It still can be found in some stores in Appalachia. Chewing tobacco was popular in both the North and South among soldiers and farmers prior to, during, and after the Civil War. Spittoons could be found in many public buildings, both in urban and rural America. Today the spittoon is an antique. Periodontal disease and oral cancers are more commonly found in tobacco chewers.

Bidis

Bidis are cheap cigarettes made from inferior tobacco products and laced with flavors such as chocolate, vanilla, and strawberry. Bidis come from Asia, particularly poverty-stricken India where they are very popular. Bidis can be found in convenience stores and gas stations across the United States and have gained popularity among American teens because of their sweet, aromatic flavors.

Hookahs

Tall water pipes (hookahs) have been used for centuries in the Middle East and in South Asia. They have recently gained popularity among American college students. Hookah tobacco is soaked in molasses and mixed with pulp from various fruits, such as mint, mango, or apples. It is smoked communally, using disposable mouthpieces. There remains a myth among some people that water pipe smoking is safer than smoking cigarettes. Smoking from a hookah may be more dangerous than traditional forms of smoking. The tobacco contains more tar and nicotine than cigarettes and also may contain heavy metals. Additionally, hookah smoke produces

The Basics

more carbon monoxide than cigarette smoke because of the charcoal used to heat the tobacco. The hookah user may inhale as much smoke during a single hookah session as a cigarette smoker does after smoking 100 cigarettes. Another concern is that communal smoking creates a risk for the spread of communicable diseases, including herpes and tuberculosis.

5. Is tobacco a drug?

There is no single, precise definition for a drug, but generally speaking, a drug is defined as a compound that, when ingested, alters bodily function in some manner. Surprisingly, it was not until 1996 that the Food and Drug Administration (FDA) declared nicotine a drug and thus attempted unsuccessfully to bring it under its jurisdiction (see question 19 for more information). This unusual fact has to do with the differences that exist between various definitions of drug. There are definitions that are chemical, biological, medical, cultural, and legal. With respect to the legal definition, defining nicotine as a drug changes the laws that regulate its distribution and use. This is why, even though coffee and cocoa are technically drugs, they are not drugs under the legal definition. The role of the FDA is to ensure the "purity, safety, and effectiveness of drugs and the 'devices' used to deliver drugs." Nicotine is defined as a drug and the cigarette is defined as a delivery device. According to the FDA, nicotine is a drug because it stimulates the brain and enhances feelings of pleasure, thereby reinforcing its continued use by the individual. In other words, nicotine alters the functions of both the body and the brain, which meets the FDA definition of a drug. Another effect is the damage cigarettes cause to the body, notably to the lungs and cardiovascular system, often causing cancer and death. This adds to the definition and furthers the need for control by the FDA. Consequently, the FDA attempted to place restrictions on tobacco advertising and sales to minors. However, this was overturned by the Supreme Court until 2008, when Congress finally passed a law granting the FDA authority.

According to the FDA, nicotine is a drug because it stimulates the brain and enhances feelings of pleasure, thereby reinforcing its continued use by the individual.

Joseph's comment:

From my point of view, I feel that tobacco is a drug with one of the strongest levels of addiction. It keeps you in such place of denial because when I was smoking, I could not see that I was ruled by the tobacco. After quitting, I began to see that tobacco controlled every aspect of my life. Even after breaking the physical addiction, there was still more work to do on the mental addiction.

6. What are tar and nicotine?

Tar

Tar is the brown, sticky substance left at the end of a cigarette filter after it is smoked. It includes additional ingredients to give cigarettes a better flavor. The by-products of smoking these other ingredients are inhaling toxic chemicals. Tar is made up of more than 4000 chemicals; some of the more toxic chemicals include cyanide, benzene, ammonia, and methanol (wood alcohol). Tar causes the cilia in the lungs to stop functioning. *Cilia* are small protrusions (like the tentacles on sea urchins) that trap and remove foreign substances from the lungs. Tar is also carcinogenic because it alters the cell's genetic material. When the cells reproduce, new abnormal cells are created that lead to cancer.

Tar leaves a brownish-yellow film on contact. This is responsible for the brown residue that stains a smoker's teeth and fingers. It leaves stains in the environment where cigarettes are smoked (fabric, walls and ceilings, etc.). Filters were added to cigarettes in the 50s when it first became known that tars were potentially dangerous to one's health as a way of trapping and reducing their amount. Later, low-tar cigarettes were also produced with a similar thought. Cigarettes were classified as *high-tar*, *medium-tar*, and *low-tar* by the amount of tar they contained. Low-tar cigarettes are marketed as "lights."

Tar, nicotine, and carbon monoxide ceiling values (more commonly defined as **TNCO ceilings**) are international standards

TNCO (Tar, Nicotine, and Carbon Monoxide) Ceilings

The total upper value of the aerosol residue, nicotine, and carbon monoxide contents as measured by a cigarette smoking machine calibrated to ISO standards. This measure is used by countries worldwide to regulate manufactured tobacco products.

that many governments use to set limits on how tobacco companies may manufacture and market cigarettes in their countries. It is important to understand that different countries set different limits. These standards are based on smoking machines and not on human consumption. Because humans tend to modify the way they inhale cigarettes in order to make up for any lost flavor or nicotine amount, studies by the National Cancer Institute (NCI) have shown that low-tar or light cigarettes contain no health advantages over high-tar, or full-flavor cigarettes. We cover some of the more important chemicals in greater detail in Questions 12 and 13.

High-tar cigarettes contain at least 22 milligrams (mg) of tar. Medium-tar cigarettes have from 15 mg to 21 mg, and low-tar cigarettes contain 7 mg or less of tar.

Nicotine

Nicotine, which is named from the plant after its introduction to Europe by Jean Nicot, was first isolated in 1823, and synthesized in 1893. It is a chemical compound in a family of nitrogen-containing plant-based compounds collectively known as **alkaloids**. Alkaloids include many psychoactive compounds, such as cocaine, caffeine, and opium. Nicotine is found in a family of plants known as *Solanaceae*. The family is also informally known as the potato family, which includes a wide variety of common plants such as potato, tomato, eggplant, green peppers, chili peppers, paprika as well as belladonna (the deadly poisonous nightshade). Nicotine is predominantly found in tobacco, but in lesser quantities in some of the other plant family members, too. Nicotine can be found in non-solanaceous plants, such as in the leaves of the coca plant, which is more commonly known as the basis for the drug cocaine.

Nicotine is made in the roots and accumulates in the leaves. Its primary purpose is to repel bugs (insecticide) in order to protect itself. It was used for this purpose for many centuries

Alkaloids

Naturally occurring chemical compounds containing basic nitrogen atoms that are produced by a large variety of organisms, including bacteria, fungi, plants, and animals.

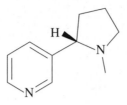

Figure 1   Molecular Structure of Nicotine

by humans as well, and nicotine derivatives continue to be widely used as insecticides to this day. It is an organic compound, which is a compound that consists predominantly of carbon and hydrogen. **Figure 1** shows the chemical structure (N stands for nitrogen).

7. How do chemicals such as nicotine work in the brain?

First, knowing how the brain works in general and how chemicals interact with neurons to alter communication between nerve cells is a good basis for understanding how the brain responds to nicotine. The brain is a complex organ comprised of gray matter and white matter. Gray matter consists of the cell bodies of neurons and other support cells. White matter consists of long tracts of **axons** that run between the neurons (like telephone lines) in order to communicate to other brain regions. **Figure 2** is an illustration of a neuron. Different areas of the brain have different functions. For example, the motor cortex controls voluntary movements, and the sensory cortex processes information from the senses (sound, sight, smell, touch, and taste). These different areas communicate with each other in an orchestrated fashion via the axons of the neurons within the areas of white matter in the brain.

The brain contains billions of neurons, which interact with each other electrochemically. This means that when a nerve is stimulated, a series of chemical events occur that in turn

Axon

That part of the neuron or nerve cell that is a long tube conducting neural signals away from the cell body.

The Basics

15

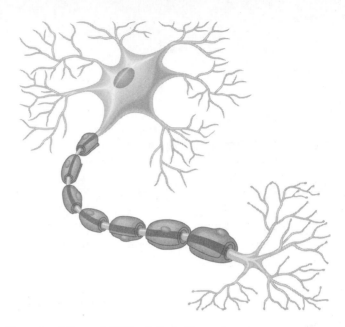

Figure 2   A Nerve Cell (Also Called a Neuron)

From D. Chiras, *Human Biology, 5th Edition.* © 2005, Jones and Bartlett LLC.

Neurotransmitters

Chemicals released by nerves that communicate with other nerves causing electrochemical changes in those nerves to continue to propagate a signal.

create an electrical impulse. The resulting impulse is repeated down the nerve length (known as the axon) and causes a release of chemicals called **neurotransmitters** into a space between the stimulated nerve and the nerve it wishes to communicate with, known as the synapse (**Figure 3**). The neurotransmitters interact with receptors on the second nerve, either stimulating them or inhibiting them. The interaction between the neurotransmitters and receptors can be likened to a key interacting with a lock. The neurotransmitter acts as the key and engages the receptor to unlock, causing it to open. This opening is really a structural change within the receptor on the second nerve that either causes that nerve to fire or not to fire. Brain activity is the result of an orchestrated series of nerves firing or not firing in binary fashion. It is much like a computer where very complicated processes begin as a series of ones or zeros (on or off, fire or don't fire).

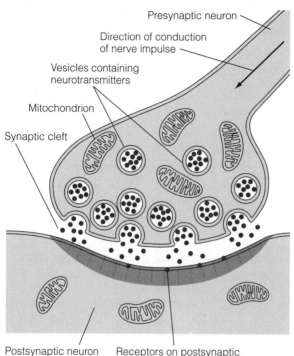

Figure 3   Synaptic Transmission

From D. Chiras, *Human Biology, 5th Edition*. © 2005, Jones and Bartlett LLC.

After the nerve fires, thereby releasing neurotransmitters into the synaptic cleft, the neurotransmitters must be removed from the area in order to turn the signal off. There are two ways these chemicals can be removed in order to turn the signal off. The first is by destroying the chemical through the use of another chemical known as an **enzyme** with that specific purpose in mind. The second is by pumping the chemical back up into the nerve that released it by utilizing another special chemical known as a transporter or **transport pump**. The process of pumping chemicals back into the nerve is known as **reuptake**. It is important to understand these basic principles of neurophysiology because all psychoactive

The Basics

Enzyme

A biological molecule that catalyzes or accelerates a chemical reaction. Most enzymes are proteins.

Transport Pump

A protein involved in reuptake of neurotransmitters.

Reuptake

A transporter protein located presynaptically that serves to transport a neurotransmitter back up into the neuron, essentially ending transmission between two nerves.

Nicotinic Receptors

Short for nicotinic acetylcholine receptors, they form ion-gated channels in certain neurons. They are located at the neuromuscular junction as well as on the postganglionic sympathetic and parasympathetic nervous system in the body. Stimulation of these receptors causes muscle contraction.

compounds, whether neurotransmitters, hormones, medications, addictive drugs, or nicotine, involve one or more of these mechanisms. The differences between their effects stem from the particular receptor and neurotransmitter system with which they interact. Nicotine, like many neurotransmitters, targets a specific neurotransmitter or receptor system known as the nicotinic acetylcholine receptor. Just as nicotine targets **nicotinic receptors**, opiates target opiate receptors and marijuana targets marijuana receptors (referred to as cannabinoid receptors), which means the body produces chemicals with similar activity as their ingested cousins.

8. Where does nicotine act on the nervous system?

In order to properly answer this question, it's good to have a brief overview of the nervous system (**Figure 4**). The nervous system can be subdivided into two broad categories, the central nervous system (CNS) and the peripheral nervous system (PNS). Nicotine receptors are found in both the CNS and PNS. The CNS includes the brain and the spinal column, both of which are protected by bone; the PNS includes all the nerves that branch out from the CNS and end at the organs of the body. Additionally, the PNS can be further subdivided into the somatic (or voluntary nervous system) and the autonomic (or involuntary nervous system). We first discuss the PNS and the location of nicotine receptors there. Next, we'll talk about the CNS, most notably the brain, and what role nicotine receptors play there.

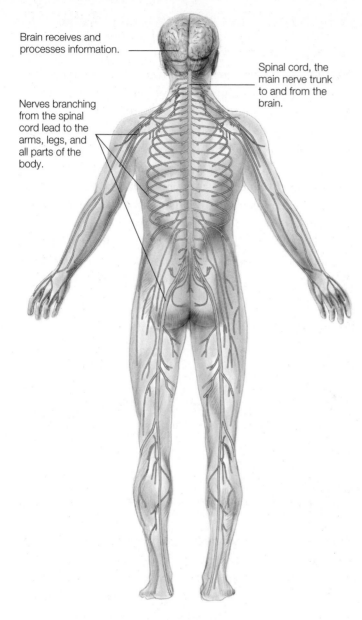

Brain receives and processes information.

Spinal cord, the main nerve trunk to and from the brain.

Nerves branching from the spinal cord lead to the arms, legs, and all parts of the body.

The Basics

Figure 4   The Central Nervous System

From D. Chiras, *Human Biology, 5th Edition.* © 2005, Jones and Bartlett LLC.

Peripheral Nervous System (PNS)

Somatic Nervous System

The somatic nervous system is that part of the PNS that plays a role in the voluntary movement of skeletal muscle (as opposed to the autonomic or involuntary nervous system, which will be discussed later). Electrochemical signals begin at the motor cortex of the CNS, are transmitted down the spinal column, and ultimately through the PNS, terminating at their respective muscles via the neuromuscular junction. The **neuromuscular junction** is the point at which the nerves end and their electrochemical communication is converted into a release of the neurotransmitter **acetylcholine**, which then prompts the muscles to move. This occurs by acetylcholine binding to the nicotinic acetylcholine receptors.

Autonomic Nervous System

The autonomic nervous system is yet further subdivided into two broad categories: (1) the sympathetic nervous system, responsible for the "fight or flight" response and (2) the parasympathetic nervous system, responsible for the "rest and restoration" response. **Figure 5** illustrates the autonomic nervous system.

Sympathetic Nervous System

The fight or flight response causes a sudden change in bodily functions as a result of a perceived threat in the environment. It diverts blood away from the digestive organs and skin to the muscles, raises the heart rate and blood pressure, dilates the airways of the lungs, and promotes alertness. In other words, it readies the body to react to the perceived threat so that it can either fight or flee from the threat.

These actions occur with the aid of the hormone **epinephrine** (also known as adrenalin because it comes from the adrenal glands) and the neurotransmitter norepinephrine in

---

Neuromuscular Junction

The junction of the axon terminal of a motor neuron with the muscle fiber responsible for ultimately causing the muscle to contract.

Acetylcholine

A neurotransmitter found in both the peripheral nervous system (PNS) and the central nervous system (CNS). In the PNS, it is involved in both muscle contraction as well as that part of the involuntary nervous system involved with "rest and restoration." In the CNS, it is involved with memory function.

Epinephrine

(Also known as the hormone adrenaline.) A catecholamine derived from tyrosine, an amino acid, which is produced in the adrenal medulla and released into the bloodstream to activate the "fight or flight" response via the sympathetic nervous system.

the sympathetic nervous system. (Finally, the neurotransmitter dopamine is also activated but in a more limited manner.) All of these chemicals are collectively known as **catecholamines**. Norepinephrine and epinephrine bind to adrenergic receptors (also known as adrenoreceptors after adrenalin). There are two broad subtypes of adrenoreceptors known as alpha- and beta-adrenergic receptors, and many of the blood pressure medications prescribed today act at these sites by blocking them in order to lower blood pressure.

The sympathetic nervous system is also activated by the neurotransmitter acetylcholine. However acetylcholine's role is more complicated and indirect in that it stimulates receptors that are located between nerve bundles known as **ganglion** (Figure 5). The ganglion are located parallel between the

Catecholamines

Chemicals used as neurotransmitters and produced from the amino acid tyrosine. They include epinephrine, norepinephrine, and dopamine, all of which are produced in the brain as well as in the adrenal medulla, which is part of the sympathetic nervous system.

The Basics

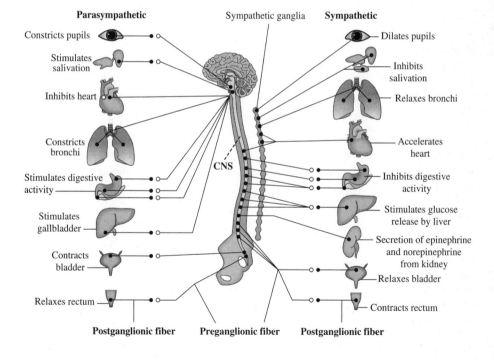

Figure 5   Autonomic Nervous System

Ganglion

A mass of tissue, generally nervous, which provides relay points and intermediary connections between different neurological structures in the body, such as the peripheral and central nervous systems.

Preganglionic

The end of the central nervous system as it is communicating with the autonomic nervous system, which is part of the peripheral nervous system.

Postganglionic

The beginning of the autonomic nervous system, which transmits from the central nervous system to the various organs. Nicotinic receptors are located here.

Adrenal medulla

The central part of the adrenal gland surrounded by the adrenal cortex. It produces adrenalin (also known as epinephrine), norepinephrine, and dopamine.

spinal cord and the organs in the illustration, which are junctions between the nerves coming from the CNS (also known as **preganglionic**) to the PNS, with peripheral nerves going to their respective organs (also known as **postganglionic**). As stated earlier, at the end organ sites, instead of acetylcholine, epinephrine and norepinephrine act as the neurotransmitters. The only exceptions to that are the **adrenal medulla**, which can be considered like a giant ganglion, and the sweat glands, which also respond to acetylcholine. As a reminder, while not directly part of the sympathetic nervous system, acetylcholine is also the neurotransmitter of the somatic nervous system as mentioned previously. Acetylcholine controls voluntary muscles, causing them to react.

Parasympathetic Nervous System

The rest and restoration response of the parasympathetic nervous system has the opposite effect of the sympathetic nervous system's fight or flight response. This response diverts blood from the muscles to the digestive organs and skin, lowers the heart rate and blood pressure, constricts the airways of the lungs, and promotes sleep. Unlike the sympathetic nervous system, all of these actions are mediated by only one neurotransmitter, acetylcholine, both at the ganglion and at the terminal endings of the organ systems. Moving blood from the muscles to the other organs aids in digestion and promotes rest so that the body can rejuvenate and prepare for the next threat. However, the ganglionic acetylcholine receptors differ from the terminal end organ acetylcholine receptors.

Acetylcholine Receptor Subtypes

There are two broadly different acetylcholine receptors: muscarinic and nicotinic acetylcholine receptors. They are named after the major chemical that stimulates each of them: Acetylcholine stimulates both receptors while muscarine stimulates only **muscarinic** acetylcholine receptors, and nicotine stimulates nicotinic acetylcholine receptors. Nicotinic acetylcholine receptors are located at multiple sites. These include the entire ganglion in the sympathetic and parasympathetic nervous system, the adrenal medulla and the sweat glands, which are also part of the sympathetic nervous system, and finally at the neuromuscular junction of the somatic nervous system. Muscarinic acetylcholine receptors are located at the end organ sites of the parasympathetic nervous system, such as the smooth muscles of the gastrointestinal tract, bladder, heart, and blood vessels.

Each of these two acetylcholine receptors has several subtypes, whose functions vary in response to stimulation from acetylcholine. Each receptor subtype responds to different chemicals as well as to acetylcholine, and either nicotine or muscarine (hence the name nicotinic receptor and muscarinic receptor). These receptors are further classified by subtypes in a very complex manner that allows for further sub-specialization. For nicotine, there are two broad subtypes: neuronal-type and muscle-type. They are further subdivided by their molecular make-up and their genetic similarities. Some are located only in the brain, some in the autonomic ganglia, and others only at the neuromuscular junction, the point at which the somatic nerves terminate on skeletal muscle. In total, nicotinic receptors contain 4 subfamilies comprising 17 subunits. This further sub-specialization allows the nicotinic receptor subtypes to differ in their response to various chemicals at muscle tissues and nervous tissues. Many of the historical toxins from plants and animals act on either the muscarinic receptor types, such as atropine from the deadly nightshade, or the nicotinic receptor types, such as curare (found on the skin of frogs and used in poison darts), and **alpha-bungarotoxin** (found in snake venom), which act at the neuromuscular junction leading to paralysis. **Figure 6** shows the nicotine receptor.

Central Nervous System (CNS)

Acetylcholine's role is also multiple in the CNS. It principally acts as a **neuromodulator,** which means that it affects many other neurotransmitter systems to coordinate their activity as

Muscarinic

Referring to muscarine, a chemical that stimulates acetylcholine receptors, located in the brain and the parasympathetic nervous system.

Alpha-bungarotoxin

A snake venom that binds irreversibly to nicotinic acetylcholine receptors at the neuromuscular junction, causing paralysis and death.

Neuromodulator

A process in which one neuron uses different neurotransmitters to connect to several neurons, as opposed to direct synaptic transmission where one neuron directly reaches another neuron.

The Basics

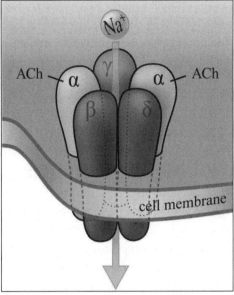

Figure 6   A Schematic Illustration of an Acetylcholine Receptor

Illustration by Giovanni Maki. © 2004 Tabitha M. Powledge. (*PLoS Biol.* 2004 November; 2(11): e404. Published online 2004 November 16. doi: 10.1371/journal.pbio.0020404.)

Anticholinergic

A substance that blocks the effects of acetylcholine in the nervous system.

Acetylcholin-esterase

An enzyme that breaks down acetylcholine, rendering it inactive. Blocking this enzyme leads to a relative increase in acetylcholine.

Limbic areas

A set of brain structures that includes the hippocampus, amygdala, and anterior thalamic nuclei that support a variety of functions including emotion, behavior, and long-term memory. These structures are closely associated with the olfactory structures.

well. It plays a very important role in attention, learning, and memory. Many areas of the brain are involved in learning and memory. Patients with Alzheimer's disease lose acetylcholine nerves at a faster rate than normal, partly explaining the loss of learning and memory as a symptom of the disease. Any chemical that can pass into the brain and block acetylcholine receptors (known as an **anticholinergic**) therefore can negatively impact learning and memory. Many of the new medications for Alzheimer's disease work by blocking the enzyme responsible for breaking down acetylcholine, known as **acetylcholinesterase**. These acetylcholinesterase inhibitors cause an increase in the amount of acetylcholine and thus improve learning and memory. Acetylcholine also modulates the experience of pain and pleasure in the centers of the brain, known as the **limbic areas**. Clearly, there is a strong link between these centers, our emotional life, and the memory centers because the strongest memories are usually elicited by strong emotions linked to pleasure and pain. Because the limbic area is the area of pleasure, this is predominantly part of the "reward system" of the brain. Acetylcholine nicotinic receptors act in this area to modulate another neurotransmitter—**dopamine**—which appears to play an important role in addiction, in addition to its role in attention and alertness.

Finally, acetylcholine plays a role in appetite regulation, particularly in areas of the brain such as the **hypothalamus**, which is one of the principle centers acting to regulate appetite. Nicotinic acetylcholine stimulation suppresses appetite. Many anticholinergic medications have the opposite effect and can stimulate appetite. (Question 91 has more information about the link between nicotine and appetite.)

9. What are the physiological effects of nicotine?

Now that we have a general outline of the neuroanatomy of acetylcholine, and about where nicotine receptors are and the general impact they have on the body, we are more informed about nicotine's physiological effects (Questions 7 and 8). Obviously, this is very complicated, as there are many receptor subtypes. Different locations in the body utilize different subtypes.

First, let's focus on the sympathetic nervous system locations: Those include (1) the adrenal medulla, considered essentially to be its own sympathetic ganglion, which releases the hormone adrenalin (along with other hormones); (2) the neuromuscular junction, which causes the skeletal muscles to activate; and finally, (3) the sweat glands on the skin. Thus, nicotine plays a role in releasing adrenalin, activating skeletal muscle, and keeping the body temperature regulated when it exerts itself. While skeletal muscles respond to nicotine, its direct impact is relatively insignificant at the doses normally ingested in the form of cigarette smoke. However, muscle twitching can occur in an overdose. Nicotine's impact on

The Basics

Dopamine

One of the brain's major neurotransmitters, dopamine is responsible for attention, alertness, decision making, reward, pleasure, and elevated mood.

Hypothalamus

Located below the thalamus, just above the brain stem, this part of the brain links the nervous system to the endocrine system via the pituitary gland.

muscles is not why it is used nor is it related to its addictive potential. Here we can see how nicotine is associated with energy and action.

Nicotine also plays a role in the parasympathetic nervous system, principally through its actions on the autonomic ganglion, which stimulates the parasympathetic nervous system and, as a result, its terminal actions on various organ systems involved in rest and restoration. These effects include activation of the gut, slowing of the heart, relaxation of the blood vessels, and stimulation of the sex organs. Acetylcholine is responsible for arousal and erection via the parasympathetic nervous system, while epinephrine is responsible for orgasm and ejaculation via the sympathetic nervous system, both of which respond to nicotine. In early history, nicotine was thought to be an aphrodisiac, and this explains why. **Table 1** outlines the various responses that occur in the major organs receiving input from the autonomic nervous system.

10. What are the psychological effects of nicotine?

In the brain, nicotine acts on the nicotinic acetylcholine receptors, which in turn act as neuromodulators that affect the actions of many other neurotransmitters. These include: acetylcholine, norepinephrine, epinephrine, dopamine, serotonin, and endorphins. The psychological effects of these various neurotransmitters include improved attention, concentration, learning and memory, in addition to enhanced pleasure, diminished pain response, and decreased anxiety.

Thus, nicotine offers a seeming paradox that cannot be duplicated by any other drug available. This paradox is a relaxed alertness, which only further adds to its appeal as a drug. It appears that smokers also can modify one effect over the other by changing the way they inhale. Studies have shown that smokers who wish to achieve a stimulating effect take short quick puffs, which produce a low level of blood nicotine thereby stimulating nerve transmission.

Table 1   Responses of Major Organs to Autonomic Nerve Impulses

Organ	Sympathetic Stimulation (preganglionic nicotinic acetylcholine, postganglionic adrenergic)	Parasympathetic Stimulation (preganglionic nicotinic, postganglionic muscarinic acetylcholine)
Heart	Increased heart rate	Decreased heart rate
	Increased force of contraction	Decreased force of contraction
	Increased conduction velocity	Decreased conduction velocity
Arteries	Constriction	Dilation
	Dilation	
Veins	Constriction	
	Dilation	
Lungs	Bronchial muscle relaxation	Bronchial muscle contraction
		Increased bronchial gland secretions
Gastro-intestinal tract	Decreased motility	Increased motility
	Contraction of sphincters	Relaxation of sphincters
Liver	Glycogen breakdown	Glycogen synthesis
	Glucose synthesis	
	Lipid breakdown	
Kidney	Renin secretion	
Bladder	Relaxation	Contraction
	Contraction of sphincter	Relaxation of sphincter
Uterus	Contraction of pregnant uterus	
	Relaxation of pregnant and non-pregnant uterus	
Eye	Dilates pupil	Constricts pupil
		Increased secretions
Salivary glands	Viscous salivary secretions	Watery salivary secretions

Additionally, it appears that at low doses, nicotine modulates the actions of norepinephrine and dopamine in the brain. This further enhances attention and concentration in a manner similar to traditional stimulants. At higher doses, nicotine also modulates the effects of serotonin opiate activity, which produces a relaxed, calming effect. (Questions 32 and 83 have more information about the effects of nicotine.)

11. How dangerous is nicotine?

As stated in Question 10, nicotine can act as a stimulant or as a sedative. Both of these effects are dose-dependent. But at higher doses, nicotine can cause hallucinations, or worse. Consider the fact that nicotine is an insecticide. Most insecticides are *neurotoxic*. This means they target the nervous system of insects in order to kill them. Many chemicals used for chemical warfare in World War I were neurotoxins first developed as insecticides, and these are still used as insecticides today. Many plant and animal poisons are neurotoxins. So the question of whether or not nicotine is dangerous is a matter of dosing. When considering dosing, you should also consider potency—that is, how much of the drug is required to achieve its desired effect, and how much of the drug is required to kill you. This is known in medicine as the therapeutic window; the narrower the therapeutic window, the more dangerous the drug. Nicotine is probably the most toxic substance regularly used by humans recreationally. It is far more toxic than even cocaine, which has been publicized in the media because of a number of famous people who have died from accidental overdose as well as stories of so-called mules, or people who died trying to smuggle the drug into the country. They do this by placing it in balloons and swallowing it and receive a lethal dose should a balloon burst. It takes about 600 mg of cocaine to kill a man. It takes only about a tenth of that amount—60 mg—of nicotine to kill a man. A typical cigarette contains anywhere from 0.5 to 2 mg of nicotine. A line of cocaine contains about 35 to 40 mg of cocaine, depending upon its purity.

Nicotine is probably the most toxic substance regularly used by humans recreationally.

12. *What are some of the important chemicals making up tar? How do these chemicals affect the brain and the body?*

More than 4,000 chemicals, including 200 poisons such as DDT, ammonia, arsenic, formaldehyde, and carbon monoxide, are found in tobacco. Some of these chemicals are native to the plant while others have been added to improve the odor and dampen the harshness of smoking so that the overall smoking experience is improved. Sugars and honey have been added to cigarettes to sweeten their taste, while ammonia speeds the absorption of nicotine into the bloodstream and ultimately to smokers' brains. Coca is sometimes added as a **bronchodilator**, which means it opens up the airways for faster delivery.

Botanical additives are extracts derived from various plants and herbs used to enhance the flavor, but they also may have pharmacological effects. For example, some pharmacological effects include anesthetic, antibacterial, anti-cancer, anti-inflammatory, anti-fungal, and anti-viral properties. However, these beneficial properties are lost once the herbs are burned and inhaled. Menthol is also added to cigarettes for taste. Menthol has numbing properties, which allows for a deeper inhalation of smoke. Many tobacco additives can contribute to allergic reactions that may also alter the body's cells, predisposing them to cancers and other ailments. The purpose of the additives is to improve the taste and smell of cigarettes in order to keep people smoking. **Table 2** lists the major ingredients, what products they are more commonly found in, and their effects on the body.

Bronchodilator

A drug or chemical that relaxes the smooth muscle of the bronchi and bronchioles to open the airways, allowing more air to reach the lungs. Commonly prescribed in patients with airway diseases such as asthma and COPD.

Table 2   Ingredients in Cigarette Smoke and Their Adverse Effects

Ingredient	Common Product	Adverse Effect
Cadmium	Oil paint	Teeth stains
Hydrogen cyanide	Poison	Respiratory problems
Carbon monoxide	Car exhaust	Blocks oxygen in blood
Vinyl chloride	Garbage bags	Reynaud-like syndrome
Toluene	Embalmer's glue	Inflamed, cracked skin
Benzene	Rubber cement	Drowsiness, headache, nausea
Naphthalene	Paint pigment	Headache, confusion
Arsenic	Ant poison	Prickly sensation in hands and feet

13. What are the chemicals in tar that are carcinogenic, and how do they cause cancer?

There are over 19 known chemicals in cigarettes that cause cancer. The most prominent of these are found in two groups: organic carcinogens and radioactive carcinogens. The organic carcinogens include polynuclear aromatic hydrocarbons, acrolein, and nitrosamines. The radioactive carcinogens comprise lead-210 and polonium-210, both of which decay into other radioactive carcinogens.

The first and most prominent polynuclear aromatic hydrocarbon identified was **benzopyrene**. Benzopyrene is metabolized into another chemical and permanently attaches to DNA (see Question 14), either killing the cell or leading to genetic mutation, which can transform it into a cancer cell. A cancer cell doesn't reproduce and die naturally, but reproduces rapidly and will replace cells in a tissue, organ, and, if left unchecked, an entire body system before killing the organism.

Benzopyrene

A class of anti-anxiety medications that include the drugs commonly known as Valium and Xanax.

Acrolein, the other chemical, gives cigarette smoke its characteristic odor and is irritating to the nose and lungs. It also binds permanently to DNA. Acrolein is 1000 times greater in cigarette smoke than benzopyrene. **Nitrosamines** are a group of compounds found in cigarette smoke but not in uncured tobacco leaves. They form as a result of curing. Nitrosamines also are produced by some foods through grilling and frying, and there is a correlation between the amounts of certain foods (such as grilled red meats) that are eaten and incidence of colon cancer. The radioactive elements in tobacco are a result of their natural exposure to minerals in the soil, so their content varies widely with the soil content. Whether or not these radioactive chemicals are found in sufficient quantities to cause cancer remains open to debate. Some researchers argue that they are of sufficient quantity to account for most of the lung cancer related to smoking.

14. How does smoking alter DNA?

Deoxyribonucleic acid (DNA) is the molecular basis of heredity located in the cell nuclei. DNA is the material that makes up a person's genes, which is necessary for the construction, organization, and function of living cells, tissues, organs, and organisms. Many of humans' most basic traits are influenced by DNA to varying degrees, such as height, weight, types of intellectual and athletic skills, and personality traits. Additionally, DNA can influence the susceptibility to develop certain diseases, including addiction and cancer. No heritability from DNA is one-to-one. In other words, even where DNA plays a large role in the inheritance of a particular trait, such as eye and skin color, it is never 100%. DNA essentially sets boundaries between two extremes, but where a trait ultimately falls within those boundaries, in large part will be determined by one's environment. Environmental influences therefore still alter any particular trait. Given that even traits that are "hardwired" into DNA can change, when we talk about the traits that are less hardwired (such as the susceptibility to

---

The Basics

Arcolein

Responsible for the gummy yellowish residue and acrid smell from burning cigarettes. It is considered carcinogenic and is toxic to the skin. It was used in chemical warfare during World War I.

Nitrosamines

Nitrosamines are found in many foods, including beer, fish, and also in meat and cheese products preserved with nitrite pickling salt. They are also produced from grilling and frying food as well as from burning tobacco. Carcinogenic in a wide variety of animal species, a feature suggesting that they may also be cancer-causing in humans.

developing cancer or addiction), DNA is less of an influence than environment.

The term *environment* requires some discussion. Most people think of environment in terms of inheritance as the immediate surroundings. These may be family, geography, community, culture, and nationality. But environment also includes physical characteristics, from microscopic changes surrounding a cell to macroscopic changes such as air and water quality, and diet. Scientists are increasingly interested in how tobacco affects the micro-environment of the cell. They want to know what causes the DNA to change (or mutate) as a result of that environmental change. It is this idea that leads scientists to study all types of diet and air and water qualities in order to understand better how they impact the body and the cells more directly.

Smoking's impact on DNA is reciprocal. In other words, there are genetic factors that influence one's response to tobacco and tobacco in turn influences one's genes by altering them through genetic mutation. This impact is threefold:

1. Individuals can be genetically more susceptible to becoming addicted to tobacco.

2. Individuals can be genetically more susceptible to the various diseases tobacco causes.

3. Tobacco itself can directly alter DNA and cause the cell to mutate.

Three separate studies have identified a genetic link between the susceptibility to become addicted and increasing the likelihood of developing lung cancer by up to 80%. These genetic variations involve a region on chromosome 15, which codes for the nicotine receptors. Possessing a single copy of the mutation increases the risk of developing lung cancer by 30%. Possessing two copies increases the risk by 80%. Several studies have concluded that smoking damages the DNA in the cells, causing carcinogenic changes that contribute to the risk of developing cancer. Over 19 primary carcinogens have been identified in tobacco smoke, of which the major constituents were discussed previously in Question 13.

15. What is meant by a "safe" cigarette?

A "safe" cigarette is one that has been modified in such a manner as to significantly reduce the amount of tar and nicotine delivered to the body. This reduction is thought to make cigarettes safer to use. Modifications include the introduction of filters but also can include chemical modification of the tobacco. Although once advertised as safer, cigarette filters actually do not make cigarette smoking safer. Filters, low-tar and nicotine cigarettes, and mentholated cigarettes are not any safer than unfiltered, regular tobacco cigarettes. In an effort to address smokers' fears about the detrimental effects of smoking, the tobacco companies first introduced filtered cigarettes, and later low-tar and nicotine cigarettes (otherwise known as "light") and mentholated cigarettes to the public. Tar and nicotine content was tested by using smoking machines, which did not alter the inhalation of tobacco smoke. However, because smokers alter the way they smoke as a result of these modifications, namely, inhaling more deeply in order to make up for the loss in flavor and nicotine dose, in the end it became nothing more than an advertising gimmick, giving customers a false sense of security.

16. What is meant by "tobacco is a gateway drug"?

A gateway is an entrance to a new and usually unexplored area. With respect to drugs, a gateway drug is one that opens the door to the possibility of using other drugs in addition to that first drug. It is also a drug that one desires to combine with other drugs, such as drinking alcohol or coffee with smoking cigarettes. Tobacco is more often the first drug used by young people, who then, by virtue of their positive experience with it, may enter a sequential process of other drug use and experimentation. These other drugs include alcohol, marijuana, and sometimes "harder" drugs, such as cocaine and heroin. According to the *Surgeon General's Report*, 12- to 17-year-old teens, who stated that they were smokers, were three times more likely to use alcohol, eight times more likely to smoke marijuana, and twenty-two times more likely to use cocaine, than their nonsmoking peers. Adolescents who smoke are also more likely to engage in other risky behaviors. (More about the *Surgeon General's Report* is in Question 21.)

In a study that examined tobacco and drug cravings, it was found that there is a connection between tobacco smoking and illicit drug use. There is a correlation between the number of cigarettes that a person smokes and the likelihood he or she will use illegal drugs, suggesting that nicotine and other substances may share similar brain pathways that reinforce the cravings for each drug. The results of teen surveys and research studies demonstrating teen use of cigarettes and other drugs strongly support the idea that cigarettes are a "gateway drug" that can lead to other drug use.

17. What effects does the Internet have on the tobacco industry and cigarette sales and on teen smoking?

The Internet circumvents four areas of government control over the sale and distribution of tobacco: (1) restricting sales to minors; (2) raising taxes to dissuade use and apply additional revenue to the healthcare costs of continued use; (3) restriction of advertising, marketing, and promotion; and (4), fostering public disapproval of the tobacco industry and its products. The Internet has become a major player in reversing all four areas both in the United States and around the world. Recently, cigarette sales have increased because people of all ages have easy access to cheaper tobacco products via the Internet. A quick Google search finds close to 700,000 cigarette Web sites that offer tax-free cigarettes to anyone, regardless of age, with access to a computer and electronic payment.

Internet sales to minors have increased because of the ability of teenagers to buy cheap cigarettes from Web sites without federal or state oversight. A recent survey found that students under 18 were able to buy cigarettes (including Marlboro Lights and Bidis) by the carton online without either being asked their age or requiring proof of their age. Many Internet Web sites that sell different types of tobacco products do not list age restrictions, and few of them have the Surgeon General's warning labels. Only one Web site used 21 years as the required age to buy cigarettes. Verification of age is by self-report (http://www.cigarettes-below-cost.com). A study commissioned by *Hot Wired*, the online version of *Hot Wired* magazine, found that 37% of Americans who buy cigarettes online are younger than 18 years of age. Only a few sites use a more rigorous approach such as verifying the buyer's age by a driver's license number or a photo ID.

Internet sales to minors have increased because of the ability of teenagers to buy cheap cigarettes from Web sites without federal or state oversight.

The Basics

18. What is the legal age to smoke?

The legal age to smoke is currently set by each state. In most states the legal age is 18. In 2002, agreements were made by Exxon Mobil and Walgreen Corporations with the states not to sell cigarettes to underage smokers. The corporations agreed to:

- Require that no one under the legal age of 18 is permitted to purchase smoking paraphernalia including cigarettes, lighters, matches, cigarette papers, and pipes.

- Be aware that youth access to tobacco shall be given comparable treatment as underage access to alcohol.

- Require that store personnel make every reasonable effort to cooperate in the enforcement of the state's youth access laws.

- Prohibit the sale of single cigarettes or "Kiddie Packs" (under 20 cigarettes/pack).

- Prohibit the distribution of free samples.

- Prohibit the sale of non-tobacco products that are designed to look like tobacco products, such as bubble gum and candy cigars or cigarettes.

- Require an ID in connection with tobacco purchases and tobacco paraphernalia by persons appearing to be under the age of 27.

- Require a photo ID at the time of purchase.

- Be aware that state laws preempt federal laws, although where they are less restrictive they are ineligible for Federal Emergency Management Agency (FEMA) funding.

19. What is the mission of the FDA, especially in regard to tobacco?

Federal Drug Administration (FDA)

The Federal Agency devoted to ensuring the safety and effectiveness of all medications released in the United States.

The overall mission of the **Federal Drug Administration (FDA)** is to protect the public's health. President Roosevelt enacted a law in 1938 that established the FDA. As a government regulatory agency, the FDA is responsible for testing drugs and medical devices for quality and safety. It is responsible for the manufacturing, labeling, advertising, and marketing of drugs and other products, to ensure their efficacy and safety. It is responsible for three types of drugs: prescription drugs, generic drugs, and over-the-counter drugs. The FDA provides approval for advertising and marketing new drugs. It also regulates food and cosmetics, animal food, dietary supplements, biological goods, and blood products according to a set of published standards, which are enforced by inspections of laboratories, factories, and other facilities. The law establishing the FDA brought products that affect the public's health under federal regulatory authority and public scrutiny.

Until Congress passed a law in 2008, the FDA had no jurisdiction over tobacco. While Congress has passed tobacco regulations six times in its history, it had never explicitly given the FDA any direct authority over tobacco. In 1996, the FDA attempted to assert authority to regulate tobacco advertising to minors, and to oversee the warning labels on tobacco products by declaring that nicotine was a drug and cigarettes were drug delivery devices. However, in 2000, the Supreme Court denied the FDA's authority. The arguments pro and con centered on the fact that Congress had never explicitly stated that the FDA had authority over tobacco. Did the FDA need Congress to pass a law granting it special authority over tobacco, or had that authority always been with the FDA, even though it had never acted on it? Given the fact that for fifty years preceding the 1996 FDA assertion, it itself had explicitly denied that Congress had ever granted it authority over tobacco, the FDA could not now suddenly claim the opposite. In 2007, the Surgeon General, in an interview, endorsed the idea that the FDA not involve itself in the regulation of tobacco because the FDA was involved in the business of health promotion. Bringing it under the control of the FDA could give a false impression to the public that tobacco could be made into a safer product. In 2008 Congress finally passed a law granting this authority to the FDA.

20. What are the laws regulating tobacco?

The laws vary from county to state to nation and are not easily codified. The major areas of legislation primarily focused on attempts to regulate the distribution of tobacco. These laws included sales tax, advertising limits, age limits, and smoking bans in public places. Additionally, legislations focused on warning the public about the health risks of smoking by including warning labels and content descriptions. Finally, many laws have occurred as a result of lawsuits against the tobacco companies and not through legislation. Most laws are state laws, particularly those regarding sales tax. The general trend over the years has been to raise the sales tax on cigarettes both to make the product less desirable but also to support state healthcare funding. The taxes vary from state to state just as all sales taxes. Regionally, taxes tend to be lower in the South, the Midwest, and in parts of the Western interior.

In 1967, the Federal Communication Commission (FCC) required that all tobacco advertising on television be counterbalanced with ads warning of the health risks associated with smoking. In 1970 Congress passed The Public Health Cigarette Smoking Act, which banned all cigarette advertising on television and radio beginning on January 2, 1971. Smokeless forms of tobacco continued to be advertised on television and radio until 1986 when they were banned as well. In 2003, tobacco companies and magazine publications voluntarily agreed to eliminate tobacco advertisements from school editions of four prominent news magazines: *Time*, *Newsweek*, *People*, and *Sports Illustrated*. This came on the heels of huge class-action lawsuits against tobacco companies and was not the result of legislative acts.

On the international level, The World Health Organization (WHO) Framework Convention on Tobacco Control was adopted in 2003 and enacted in 2005. **Table 3** lists the significant provisions of the treaty that must be implemented. To date, the United States Congress has not signed the treaty.

21. *What are the* Surgeon General's Reports?

By the 1960s, there was growing pressure for the U.S. Public Health Service to take some kind of action against smoking. Several anti-smoking advocacy groups, for example, The American Lung Association and the American Heart Association, proposed to President Kennedy that he appoint a commission to study the implications of tobacco use in the United States. Luther Terry, then Surgeon General, appointed a committee to fully investigate the ongoing questions about smoking and health.

Persistent denials of a causal link between smoking and lung cancer by the tobacco industry stimulated the need to develop a consensus report. At that time, the consensus method was unprecedented in medicine. It became the model for evidence-based medicine (EBM) to help guide medical practice based on the consensus of researchers.

Table 3   The WHO Framework Convention on Tobacco Control

Topic	Measure	Articles
Demand reduction	Tax and other measures to reduce tobacco demand.	Articles 6 & 7
Passive smoking	Obligation to protect all people from exposure to tobacco smoke in indoor workplaces, public transport, and indoor public places.	Article 8
Regulation	The contents and emissions of tobacco products are to be regulated and ingredients are to be disclosed.	Article 10
Packaging and labeling	Large health warning (at least 30% of the packet cover, 50% or more recommended); deceptive labels ("mild," "light," etc.) are prohibited.	Articles 9 & 11
Awareness	Public awareness for the consequences of smoking.	Article 12
Tobacco advertising	Comprehensive ban, unless the national constitution forbids it.	Article 13
Addiction	Addiction and cessation programs.	Article 14
Smuggling	Action is required to eliminate illicit trade of tobacco products.	Article 15
Minors	Restricted sales to minors.	Article 16
Research	Tobacco-related research and information sharing among the parties.	Articles 20, 21, & 22

Committee members came from a variety of disciplines. Members included a pharmacist, a statistician, a pulmonary medicine specialist, an internist, a surgeon, a pathologist, a biologist who was a cancer specialist, a toxicologist, a chemist, a bacteriologist, an epidemiologist, and a tobacco industry spokesperson. Each member was a renowned expert in his or her field. Any individual who had already published on the issue or had publicly taken a stand was not eligible to be on the investigative committee, in order to ensure that the findings would be unbiased. The committee included smokers and nonsmokers.

After conducting a lengthy study, the committee members concluded that there is a strong link between smoking and cancer. This conclusion was based on a wide range of evidence and included both statistical and epidemiological findings. (Statistics is the study of numerical data. Epidemiology is the study of the incidence, distribution, and control of a disease found in a population.) The committee found that the death rate from cancer among male smokers was 1,000 times higher than among nonsmokers. The tobacco industry refuted the findings, calling the causal link between smoking and lung cancer a "mathematical aberration."

The *Surgeon General's Report* was released in January 1964. This was a pivotal document in the history of public health. The report provided legitimacy to the allegations that smoking is harmful. The consensus report became a model for other reports on health concerns because of the independence and the integrity of the committee members and their findings.

The next *Surgeon General's Report* focused on secondhand smoke or environmental smoke. Two major reports were issued in 1986, one from Surgeon General Koop and the other from an independent research institution, The National Academy of Sciences (NAS). Both addressed the effects of environmental smoke on nonsmokers. The two reports each confirmed the other's findings. First, mainstream smoke exhaled into the air by smokers mixed with smoke released directly from the burning end of a cigarette, and constituted approximately 85% of the nonsmoker's intake of tar and nicotine. Second, secondhand smoke also posed risks not only to vulnerable individuals, such as those with respiratory problems, but also to healthy adults and children. What had been considered an environmental nuisance became a recognized and validated risk to the health of anyone exposed to the polluted air. The conclusion was that the simplest expansive and most effective way to prevent diseases from secondhand smoke was to establish smoke-free environments, including work-sites.

22. How have the Surgeon General's Reports affected the smoking habits of Americans?

Since the publication of the *Surgeon General's Reports*, along with the mounting evidence that cigarettes were both dangerous to one's health and addictive, there has been a steady decline in smoking among Americans, including teenagers. Particularly as the dangers of environmental smoke came to the public's attention, organizations enacted rules to develop more smoke-free public facilities. Bans on smoking in public places are almost universal in the United States.

Immediately after the first year that the *Report* was made public (1964), the number of smokers declined. However, the next year the industry rebounded, reporting record sales and an increase in the per capita consumption of tobacco products. During the 1980s, cigarette consumption reached a critical point, after which the rates of smoking in the United States began a slow and progressive decline. In 1982, one-third (33%) of all adults were smokers; three years later the number had fallen to 30%. The second *Surgeon General's Report* about secondhand smoke, published in 1986, set off a cataclysmic shift away from public smoking because it adversely affected both smokers and nonsmokers. Workplace initiatives banning cigarette smoking proliferated. By the twenty-first century, smoking has declined more dramatically, and now smoking has become more of a private rather than public activity.

The second Surgeon General's Report about secondhand smoke, published in 1986, set off a cataclysmic shift away from public smoking because it adversely affected both smokers and nonsmokers.

23. What was the effect of the lobbying efforts of the flight attendants union on the rules about smoking on airlines?

The lobbying efforts of the flight attendants had a major impact on the relationship between the airline industry and the tobacco industry. Airlines changed the rules for smoking to nonsmoking on flights and in airports except in designated places.

Airplanes can be thought of as the epitome of an enclosed space, and they became the focus of debate during the late sixties. In 1971, the flight attendants complained about their working conditions because they were exposed to secondhand smoke while on their jobs. They lobbied the airline industry to ban smoking on airplanes. Both the airline industry and the tobacco industry resisted changing their policies because they feared that they would lose customers. Initially, the Civil Aeronautics Board made nonsmoking sections a requirement on all commercial flights in response to the flight attendant's demands. In 1986, the National Academy of Sciences reported that the air quality on planes was in violation of the environmental requirements for building codes and other indoor environments. Following that study, the airline industry banned all smoking on commercial flights.

PART TWO

Diagnosis

What is addiction?

How do I know if I am addicted to nicotine?

What are the physiological changes taking place
during withdrawal?

More...

24. What is addiction?

The American Society of Addiction Medicine (ASAM) defines addiction as follows:

"Addiction is a disease characterized by continuous or periodic impaired control over the use of drugs or alcohol, preoccupation with drugs or alcohol, continued use of these substances despite adverse consequences related to their use, and distortions in thinking, most notably denial."

This definition of addiction as a disease means that it has a fairly predictable course and a constellation of signs and symptoms, associated with a relatively defined pathophysiology and a scientifically validated treatment. With respect to the course of the disease, addicts typically begin by experimentation, evolve into regular but controlled use, and ultimately find themselves in periodic episodes of out of control use that causes impairment in various areas of their lives, either physically or socially. Despite these negative consequences, they continue to use.

Preoccupation with obtaining and using tobacco refers to the fact that the addictive substance plays a central part in their inner and/or outer lives, whether or not they are actively using it. Thus, maintaining abstinence is only one element in one's treatment, as the major struggle continues. Distortion in thinking includes, but is not limited to, denial. Also included are the litany of excuses for continued use, the blaming of others, particularly family members and caregivers, for one's failure to maintain abstinence, and the frequently cited identification with some other emotional problem that really needs to be addressed rather than the drug itself. The negative consequences play little if any role in modifying the continued use, which is the final aspect of addiction. From the ASAM's perspective, addiction and dependence can be used interchangeably.

Addictive behaviors may include gambling, sex, drugs, and all of the variations on those themes, which recently include the use of the Internet and involvement with pornography. From that simple definition, it appears that no biological or pathophysiological process must be invoked. The addiction may result from the involvement or the pursuit of an activity rather than on what effect the pursuit of the activity may have on the brain. How can gambling or the Internet have the same effects on the brain as nicotine or alcohol? There is no receptor specific for gambling or the Internet like there is for nicotine or alcohol. Somehow the behavior and the pursuit of an activity take on a life of their own, to the exclusion of all other activities.

25. Why has there been so much controversy regarding cigarette smoking as being addictive?

Obviously, from the perspective of tobacco companies, the financial implications regarding smoking's addictive potential were enormous. Addiction conjures up a set of images that is at best negative, at worst grossly disturbing. To associate tobacco use with heroin or cocaine addiction is neither a good marketing ploy nor generally an accurate depiction of a smoker. Smokers hold jobs, obey the law, and have normal relationships. A lesser term, such as a bad habit seems more appropriate and easier to swallow. After all, we all have bad habits, but a chronic smoker is hardly a person associated with the seedier elements of society portrayed on *Miami Vice*. A bad habit is a behavior that is acquired by frequent repetition. Although not easily broken, with a conscious effort it can be broken without withdrawal symptoms and without adverse consequences. Smoking, on the surface, seems more like this than an addiction. With increasing scientific information and greater scrutiny of tobacco companies' research into the issue and their attempt to prevent access to that research, the issue became highly politicized, eventually leading to the enormous class action lawsuits and government fines.

Joseph's comment:

Through the past couple of years, I started to feel my self-esteem was being affected by the public controversy around smoking. I tried hiding my smoking and covering my tobacco breath. I felt non-smokers looked down on me (in many respects, I agreed with them). I wasn't a bad person but an addicted person needing help.

Lisa's comment:

I attended a smoking cessation program in the early 1980s. The leader read through a virtual tirade against smokers that made the group feel like failures, people who just would not cooperate, people who simply were too lazy to perform their duty to quit smoking, and so on and so forth. The group "performed" so poorly that eventually the co-leader of the group began smoking again. Then the whole program fell apart. I was afraid to attempt another smoking cessation program for many years after that for fear of failing again.

26. Why did it take so long to determine that smoking was addictive?

Without going into the enormous details on the history of the tobacco industry and its attempts to present tobacco use simply as a matter of choice with no conclusive ill health effects, the answer lies simply in the nature of addiction and dependence. (More about the tobacco industry's strategies to conceal health risks of tobacco is in Question 95.)

Smoking does not affect behavior in any negative way in the same way as other addictions. The smoker continues to function as any nonsmoking individual would.

As noted in Question 25, tobacco smokers appear to share little in common with what most people consider addicts. The idea of a smoker struggling with a "bad habit" is more plausible on the surface. Smoking does not affect behavior in any negative way in the same way as other addictions. The smoker continues to function as any nonsmoking individual would. This occurs even when the smoker abruptly stops smoking. There are no overtly physiologically measurable effects of withdrawal. The behavioral effects are general and can be seen in anyone who forgoes a habit, whether it is considered "good" or "bad." The smoker does not end up on the streets resorting to crime to feed his or her habit, nor in the hospital in a state of acute withdrawal.

27. How can smoking be an addiction but at the same time be different from drugs we normally associate with addiction?

The answer lies in the definition of drug dependency and the confusion between this term and the terms bad habit and physiologic dependency. This subtle distinction has lead to no end of confusion regarding all forms of addiction and dependence. **Table 4** contains the *DSM-IV-TR* Criteria for Substance Dependence.

The DSM-IV-TR (*Diagnostic and Statistical Manual of Psychiatric Disorders*, 4th edition, Text Revised) is the diagnostic "gold standard" of psychiatric disorders. The writers chose to replace the term addiction with the term substance dependence in an attempt to remove the negative connotation associated with addiction. Before the substitution of the terms, dependence traditionally only referred to physiological dependency. Physiological dependency, as opposed to addiction or substance dependence, occurs with many drugs, including those not regarded as addictive, such as antihypertensive medications, anti-asthmatic medications, anticonvulsant medications, and even many over-the-counter (OTC) medications, such as aspirin. Alternatively, other drugs considered to be highly addictive are not associated with any typical physiological dependency, such as cocaine and amphetamines. Notice, after reviewing the criteria, that only three of seven of the criteria are required to make the diagnosis of substance dependence, while only two of the seven criteria refer to symptoms typically regarded as evidence of physiological dependency. Most notable are the first two criteria, which are referred to as "tolerance and withdrawal."

Table 4   Criteria for Substance Dependence According to the *Diagnostic and Statistical Manual of Psychiatric Disorders* (*DSM-IV-TR*, 4th Edition, Text Revised)

DSM-IV-TR Criteria for Substance Dependence

A maladaptive pattern of substance use, leading to clinically significant impairment or distress, as manifested by **three (or more)** of the following, occurring at any time in the same 12-month period:

1. tolerance, as defined by either of the following:

    a. a need for markedly increased amounts of the substance to achieve intoxication or desired effect

    b. markedly diminished effect with continued use of the same amount of the substance

2. withdrawal, as manifested by either of the following:

    the characteristic withdrawal syndrome for the substance

    the same (or a closely related) substance is taken to relieve or avoid withdrawal symptoms

3. the substance is often taken in larger amounts or over a longer period than was intended

4. there is a persistent desire or unsuccessful efforts to cut down or control substance use

5. a great deal of time is spent in activities necessary to obtain the substance (e.g., visiting multiple doctors or driving long distances), use the substance (e.g., chain-smoking), or recover from its effects

6. important social, occupational, or recreational activities are given up or reduced because of substance use

7. the substance use is continued despite knowledge of having a persistent or recurrent physical or psychological problem that is likely to have been caused or exacerbated by the substance (e.g., current cocaine use despite recognition of cocaine-induced depression, or continued drinking despite recognition that an ulcer was made worse by alcohol consumption)

    The diagnosis should specify "With Physiological Dependence" (either item 1 or 2 is present) or "Without Physiological Dependence" (neither item 1 nor 2 is present).

Source: Copyright © 2008 American Psychiatric Publishing, Inc. All Rights Reserved.

To reiterate, if you meet only two of any of the seven criteria, then you do not have the diagnosis. This now allows you to disconnect physiological dependency from drug dependence, reinforcing the fact that there are drugs that can cause only physiological dependency but are not addictive, and drugs that cause addiction but do not cause physiological dependency. However, is it possible to take a drug daily that is known to cause physiological dependency *and* addiction and yet still not become addicted? The answer is "yes," as long as only the first two criteria are met. A chronic pain patient, for example, who requires daily opiate medications to manage his or her pain will develop physiological dependency, but is *not* drug dependent or addicted if he or she meets only the first two criteria. Nor, for that matter, is a depressed patient who requires daily medication to function, even though antidepressant medications can cause significant withdrawal effects if stopped abruptly. Alternatively, one need not meet either of the first two criteria, but meet three of the other criteria, to be diagnosed as drug dependent, or addicted. This would include people who use drugs we normally associate with addiction, such as cocaine, but also drugs commonly argued as being non-addictive, such as marijuana and previously, tobacco. This also allows for the inclusion of behaviors such as gambling and sex, neither of which chemically alters the body. And this only compounds the confusion. Most smokers clearly report symptoms that meet the first two criteria. They report both tolerance and withdrawal symptoms. However, scientists historically defined withdrawal not by subjective reports (or symptoms) but by objective measures (or signs) such as changes in blood pressure or pulse, tremors, sweating, diarrhea, hallucinations, or other forms of grossly aberrant behavior. Smokers demonstrated none of these signs after abrupt cessation. Thus, the tobacco companies were able to successfully argue that withdrawal did not occur because there were no objective measures to demonstrate it.

These issues about the meaning of addiction remain confusing even to this day. Physicians and medical students often believe that any patient taking an opioid or benzodiazepine medication who suffers from withdrawal symptoms after abrupt discontinuation, by definition, is addicted to that medication. They also believe that the mere fact that discontinuation of antidepressant medication leads to acute withdrawal proves these medications are addictive. And yet, at the same time, those very same physicians and students would not associate all the other medications that cause physiological withdrawal as evidence of an addictive potential. The reason for this has to do with the fact that any medication having psychotropic or psychoactive effects (that is, affecting mind, emotions, or behavior) is automatically held to be morally suspect. All other medications, regardless of their risks and withdrawal effects, are alternatively perceived as morally neutral. Thus, antidepressants are thought to be addictive by some individuals while asthma medications are not. This is an example of how culture—and not scientific evidence—continues to play a large role in many physicians' and lay persons' perceptions of medicine (**Table 5**).

Table 5   Similarities and Differences Between Tobacco Addiction and Other Drug Addictions

Similarities	Differences
Compulsive use	No behavioral intoxication or adverse behavioral outcomes
Continued use despite harm	Does not cause other mental disorders
Impaired control over drug use	Giving up or reducing activities to use is rare
Tolerance	High intensity of use
Withdrawal	Little euphoria
Mediated via dopamine release	Spending lots of time in obtaining/using/recovering from effects is rare
Rapid relapse	Dependence is rare in adult non-daily users
Rapid reinstatement of dependence	Prosocial beneficial effects

28. How do I know if I am addicted to nicotine?

Because of the fact that drug dependence is distinct from physiological dependency and the fact that addiction to nicotine is not the same as addiction to heroin or cocaine, sometimes it is difficult even for those who smoke to know whether or not they are addicted to tobacco. This is particularly true, as the criteria state (see Questions 24 and 27), if a drug does not become a central activity in people's daily lives. How one decides this is largely subjective. As Mark Twain famously said, "Giving up smoking is the easiest thing in the world. I know because I've done it thousands of times."

This quote illustrates the central dilemma regarding addiction to tobacco. How can it be addictive if it is so easy to quit? Then why do you have to quit so many times before you convince yourself you are addicted? Question 32 offers a list of common nicotine withdrawal symptoms to give a clue that, at the very least, physiological dependency has occurred. Of course, as mentioned earlier, these alone are not enough to meet all of the *DSM-IV-TR* criteria of addiction. But Twain's quote captures at least one other criterion: there is a persistent desire or unsuccessful effort to cut down or control substance use. Of course, you may argue, "but I have neither a desire nor made an effort to cut down so therefore I am not addicted!" Well, aside from the mental gymnastics that addicts go through to convince themselves they are OK, consider one more criterion: the substance use is continued despite knowledge of having a persistent or recurrent physical or psychological problem that is likely to have been caused or exacerbated by the substance (for example, current cocaine use despite recognition of cocaine-induced depression, or continued drinking despite recognition that an ulcer was made worse by alcohol consumption). The physical problems resulting from smoking are by now so well documented that anyone who does not quit despite these facts meets this criterion. Yes, we all know of Grandpa who smoked from the age of 12 until he died at the age of 100. That is always a heartening story. Unfortunately, tobacco use is like Russian roulette or any other risky activity. You can still win, but you are playing against the casino, and while some individuals win, most do not; regardless, the casino always wins.

Here are some simple warning signs that you are addicted: If you smoke within 30 minutes after getting out of bed in the morning, you are probably addicted. If you cannot resist smoking even when you are ill, you are probably addicted. If you are smoking more than one pack each day, smoking more in the morning than at other times of the day, or having difficulty refraining from smoking in places that are assigned as no smoking areas, then you are probably addicted.

Lisa's comment:

When I tried to quit in the past, using the withdrawal process without any medication support, I suffered extreme depression. I kept running to the bathroom at work or out to the parking lot to cry uncontrollably. When I got home, I'd sit on the floor and cry in a fetal position. I thought something was wrong with me and beat myself up even more for not being able to function in any normal mode.

29. What is "the vicious cycle of addiction to tobacco and nicotine"?

Drug addiction follows a cycle like this: A person experiences discomfort, a sense of distress or pain, whether physical or psychological. This person drinks or tries drugs in order to temporarily relieve the discomfort. It works and the person feels better. He or she realizes he or she can deal with life better and the drugs help toward that end. Use gradually increases as the effectiveness of the drug wears off sooner after each use. As it wears off, a new feeling of discomfort associated with the drug wearing off crowds out the previous discomfort and it fades from memory. At this point, getting and using drugs becomes the primary focus. He or she can no longer control using the drug and ignores any horrible consequences associated with its use. They now have a new problem: addiction. A

If you smoke within 30 minutes after getting out of bed in the morning, you are probably addicted.

sense of shame and embarrassment causes the addict to hide his or her drug use from friends and family. This dishonesty and guilt further add to the discomfort, causing a backlash of denial and justification for continued use. In this state of mind, social isolation becomes an easy solution. But this only compounds the discomfort further.

Relationships with friends and family and job performance are impacted. The drugs replace even those outlets and become the most important thing. Ironically, the ability to get relief diminishes as one adapts to the drugs. Ever larger amounts must be taken in order to function at all. An overwhelming obsession with getting and using the drugs now supplants all other interests or activities. One is now caught in an emotional rollercoaster that actually may be mistaken for mental illness. One may seem very "up" and enthusiastic when high, and "down" (depressed) and lethargic when in withdrawal. At this point, the addict is stuck in a cycle of addiction. One faces the problem of having to pursue drugs at any cost and to attempt to appear normal to his friends, family, and employer. By now, the drugs will have changed one both physically and mentally.

While this cycle may seem extreme, particularly when distinguishing the clear differences between nicotine addiction and other addictions, it illustrates why nicotine addiction may actually be far more difficult to quit. When facing the loss of one's entire support system and one's job, it is easier to see why one would want to quit. But when such overtly huge losses are not in jeopardy, the internal justification for continued use becomes all the more powerful, even though one's health is at stake. The impact on health is gradual and insidious, taking years to occur. It does not come in a crescendo-like force the way an alcoholic's or heroin addict's life falls apart. It's easy to rationalize that the physical condition would have occurred anyway even without smoking.

So the cycle of addiction for nicotine is far more subtle, yet because of that fact it is far more powerful and tightly bound.

To read a darkly humorous account of this cycle, I refer you to a chapter called "Smoke" in Italo Svevo's novel, *Zeno's Conscience*.

Joseph's comment:

In my experience, I truly believe that tobacco and nicotine are a part of a vicious cycle both physically and psychologically. When I first started smoking, it felt like something that worked to relax me and calm me down. At that time it was also a "cool" thing to do. Within a short period of time, I went from wanting a cigarette to needing a cigarette. Even with all the information on TV and what doctors told me, it seemed like it did not matter. What I like to call the phenomena of craving had set in. Every time I tried to not smoke, the physiological and physical draw was so strong, that my self-will could not prevent me from picking up the next one.

30. Are there different "types" of smokers, for example casual smokers versus chain smokers? Are there personality or physiological differences between types of smokers?

There are both casual smokers and chain smokers. For some, a couple of puffs can lead to an addiction. Some highly addicted smokers find it almost impossible to quit while others can make the decision to quit and never miss it.

There is no consistent evidence that supports the finding that there are specific psychological or biological traits that are linked with smoking. We do know that children of parents who smoke or did smoke are at higher risk of nicotine dependence than children whose family members do not smoke.

Psychological Traits

Although some studies point to certain personality traits that contribute to the tendency to become dependent on tobacco, the influence of the social environment and culture must also be taken into consideration. Some researchers have noted that smoking is frequently associated with drug and alcohol use, lack of physical exercise, poor nutrition, anxiety, depression, risky behaviors such as not using seat belts in automobiles, and failure to follow preventive guidelines in terms of lifestyle. These behavioral traits have been considered factors that may contribute to nicotine dependence. However, there is insufficient evidence about the relationship between personality traits and smoking. Other personality patterns that have been loosely connected to smokers are hostility, aggression, and violence.

Biological Differences

Recently, scientists have identified a single genetic variant that not only contributes to a smoker's addiction but also increases the risk of developing lung cancer. Four different teams of scientists from different parts of the world reached the same conclusion—that a genetic variant on chromosome 15 is associated both with heavy smoking and a susceptibility to lung cancer. Scientists also found that smokers who inherit these genetic variations from both parents have an 80% greater chance of becoming addicted to nicotine and at some point developing lung cancer.

31. What screening tools are used to diagnose addictive smokers?

A number of screening tools have been developed. One is a modification of the alcohol screening tool known as CAGE. CAGE is an acronym for four simple questions:

1. *C*ut down: Have you ever felt the need to cut down or control your smoking but had difficulty doing so?

2. *A*nnoyed: Do you ever get annoyed or angry with people who criticize your smoking or tell you that you ought to quit?

3. *G*uilt: Have you ever felt guilty about your smoking or about something you did while smoking?

4. *E*ye-opener: Do you ever smoke within half an hour of waking up?

Another screening tool is an outline for the *DSM-IV* diagnosis of substance dependence. It is called the Four C's test:

1. Compulsion—the intensity with which the desire to use tobacco overwhelms your thoughts, feelings, and judgment.

2. Control—the degree to which you can or cannot control tobacco use once you start using.

3. Cutting down—the effects of reducing tobacco intake, that is, withdrawal symptoms.

4. Consequences—denial or acceptance of the damage caused by tobacco use.

Table 6 shows the Fagerström Test, which is a standard instrument to assess the intensity of physical addiction.

Table 6   Modified Fagerström Test for Nicotine Dependence

1. How soon after you wake up do you smoke your first cigarette?
   Within 5 minutes (3 points)
   5 to 30 minutes (2 points)
   31 to 60 minutes (1 point)
   After 60 minutes (0 points)

2. Do you find it difficult not to smoke in places where you shouldn't, such as in church or school, in a movie, at the library, on a bus, in court or in a hospital?
   Yes (1 point)
   No (0 points)

3. Which cigarette would you most hate to give up; which cigarette do you treasure the most?
   The first one in the morning (1 point)
   Any other one (0 points)

4. How many cigarettes do you smoke each day?
   10 or fewer (0 points)
   11 to 20 (1 point)
   21 to 30 (2 points)
   31 or more (3 points)

5. Do you smoke more during the first few hours after waking up than during the rest of the day?
   Yes (1 point)
   No (0 points)

6. Do you still smoke if you are so sick that you are in bed most of the day, or if you have a cold or the flu and have trouble breathing?
   Yes (1 point)
   No (0 points)

Scoring: 7 to 10 points = highly dependent; 4 to 6 points = moderately dependent; less than 4 points = minimally dependent.

Adapted with permission from Heatherton TF, Kozlowski LT, Frecker RC, Fagerström KO. The Fagerström test for nicotine dependence: a revision of the Fagerström Tolerance Questionnaire. *Br J Addict* 1991;86:1119–1127.

32. *What are the physiological changes taking place during withdrawal?*

The brain and the body, like humans, do not take kindly to abrupt changes in their environment. When the body is exposed to small daily changes, it gradually adjusts to those changes through a process known as adaptation. Adaptation is seen in many physiological processes and occurs both at the molecular level as well as at the behavioral level. It is the whole reason behind developing strength and endurance through daily graduated exercise. The muscles increase in size and develop more blood vessels in order to deal with the increasing demands being made on them. The heart enlarges and grows stronger. Oxygen is delivered more quickly and efficiently to those organ systems requiring it. Bones get stronger to handle their increasing loads. Adaptation also occurs in the brain through a process known as **neuroplasticity**. An athlete who practices daily improves technically over time. This occurs as the brain adapts and "memorizes" by "rewiring" through neuroplasticity the correct coordination of muscle movements for maximum performance. This is often referred to by trainers and coaches as muscle memory. It occurs with all motor skills that are utilized daily, from learning to walk, to driving a car, to complex activities such as athletics, playing a musical instrument, or becoming a surgeon.

When you take a drug every day, adaptation occurs in response to the drug. As stated earlier, this happens with almost all drugs, regardless of whether or not they are addictive. However, for drugs regarded as potentially addictive the adaptation is termed *tolerance*. Tolerance is both psychological as well as physiological. When a drug is abruptly withdrawn, the body cannot adjust fast enough and withdrawal symptoms occur. Those symptoms vary depending upon the drug and the receptor system involved.

Nicotine, depending on the dosing, acts as both a stimulant by activating the sympathetic nervous system, and as a sedative,

Neuroplasticity

Changes that occur in the organization of the brain as a result of experience.

Diagnosis

GABA (Gamma Amino Butyric Acid)

The brain's major inhibitory neurotransmitter. This neurotransmitter dampens all brain activity, essentially calming the brain down at every level.

Glutamate

The brain's major excitatory neurotransmitter. This neurotransmitter activates all brain activity, essentially stimulating the brain and "lifting" it up at every level.

Homeostasis

A property of most living systems, which are organized to maintain a stable, balanced state of equilibrium.

Up-Regulation

The process by which a cell increases the number of receptors to a given hormone or neurotransmitter to improve its sensitivity to this molecule. (A decrease of receptors is called down-regulation.)

by activating the parasympathetic nervous system and reducing the activity of the sympathetic nervous system through constant stimulation (see Question 8). The body's response therefore is unique. While you may feel a general sense of activation and alertness, with a rising of the heart rate and blood pressure, and a release of adrenalin, you also feel a sense of relaxation with the stimulation of the bowels and activation of the rest and restoration response in the parasympathetic nervous system. Which system is activated more than the other is dose-dependent, and people learn how to alter the dose by changing the frequency and depth of their inhalations to vary the response. In the brain, nicotine promotes alertness and pleasure, dampens pain and appetite, and creates a general sense of relaxed attention. All of these effects are mediated not only from the direct effects of nicotine, but also from nicotine's effects on other neurotransmitter systems, including dopamine, endorphins, **GABA**, **glutamate**, and norepinephrine. Dopamine and norepinephrine improve focus and concentration, while dopamine and endorphins activate the reward system and the pleasure centers in the brain. Finally, GABA and glutamate are involved in overall brain inhibition and sedation, systems that are affected by anti-anxiety drugs such as barbiturates, benzodiazepines, and alcohol. And many of these effects persist even after a single dose of nicotine has come and gone (see Question 10). Researchers found that a single nicotine dose increases norepinephrine synthesis for at least a month.

While these effects are immediate and some long lasting, over time the brain and body adapt to the repeated exposure to the drug in order to re-establish its internal balance (**homeostasis**). Repeated exposure of nicotine to the nicotine receptor causes the effects of it to become less sensitive. The body responds to this loss of sensitivity through a process known as **up-regulation**. That is, the body produces more nicotinic receptors to restore the lost balance. This leads to physiological tolerance for which the smoker now increases the amount he or she smokes to re-obtain its pleasurable effects.

When you stop smoking abruptly, these physiological changes remain and withdrawal occurs. Now there are too many exposed nicotine receptors and the opposite effects of nicotine occur: Focus and concentration are lost; headaches and sensitivity to pain occur; hunger kicks in; fatigue and insomnia set in; constipation and dry mouth ensue. Finally, general dysphoria (malaise) and a craving for nicotine occur. These physiological effects can be sustained for months to one degree or another, while the body and brain readjust to the new environment by slowly rebuilding the receptor and neurotransmitter systems back to their original number and sensitivity.

Nicotine withdrawal symptoms:

- Cravings to smoke
- Irritability, crankiness
- Insomnia
- Fatigue
- Inability to concentrate
- Headache
- Cough
- Sore throat
- Constipation, gas, stomach pain
- Dry mouth
- Sore tongue and/or gums
- Postnasal drip
- Tightness in the chest

33. How long does it take to become addicted to tobacco?

Historically, researchers believed that it took about two years of regular use before one became tobacco dependent. Regular use has been ill defined, but was generally thought of as daily smoking of even a few cigarettes. More recently, Dr. Joseph DiFranza of the University of Massachusetts published an article in September of 2007 in the journal of *Tobacco Control* in which he argued that the beginning symptoms of addiction can take hold in teenagers as rapidly as after one cigarette. Dr. DiFranza wrote a summary article about his findings in the May 2008 edition of *Scientific American* postulating a new theory of nicotine dependency based upon some startling facts he and several colleagues discovered (Appendix). They found that many teens reported becoming addicted to cigarettes rapidly, smoking as little as only a few cigarettes a week for two months. Even smokers who were not daily users experienced withdrawal symptoms. In fact, an average of only two cigarettes a week could precipitate withdrawal symptoms, making it difficult for them to stop. Researchers working with laboratory rats found that the nicotine from one cigarette occupied close to 90% of the receptors in the brain and that after only two consecutive days of exposure, up-regulation of nicotine receptors occurred. Dr. DiFranza speculates that regular tobacco use, whether it is monthly, weekly, or daily, is not because the user finds pleasure in it but really because the user is attempting to suppress withdrawal, however mild and unconscious that sensation may be.

Sensitization-Homeostasis Theory

A theory of addiction involving two complementary systems, the craving-generation system and the craving-inhibition system, which helps to explain how a person can become addicted to tobacco after only a few cigarettes.

DiFranza terms his theory the **Sensitization-Homeostasis Theory**. He believes that the direct immediate action of nicotine is purely to suppress craving due to the increased sensitization that occurs even after the first dose, which only increases with further doses. That is the sensitization part of the theory. The homeostasis part of the theory comes in when the next dose of nicotine quickly suppresses craving and restores the newly adapted homeostatic system. Thus, there are two competing systems that are generally in a natural balance: the craving-inhibition system and the craving-generation system. When one system is activated, the other responds in order to counter the activation. Nicotine activates the craving-inhibition system. The brain then attempts to restore this balance by activating the craving-generation system, prompting one to smoke again and, like a see-saw effect, these two systems are forever out of balance. The craving-generation system is usually activated via various sensory cues such as taste, sight, and smell.

Support for this theory comes from two sources. First, **functional magnetic resonance imaging (fMRI)** studies have demonstrated that various cues associated with using tobacco in smokers cause areas of their brains to light up, which are then suppressed after the person smokes. Secondly, people who relapse after three months of quitting resume smoking at about 40% of their previous levels. This number does not change regardless of whether the person resumes smoking at three months or even three years, suggesting that there is a permanent change in the brain impacting the craving-generation system.

However, former smokers don't crave cigarettes indefinitely. Eventually their craving goes away. New adaptations in the brain occur from abstinence, which work to inhibit the craving-generation system in order to restore the balance and return to homeostasis. These adaptations are unlike smokers or non-smokers and have been visualized experimentally in laboratory animals before, during, and after exposure to nicotine.

Diagnosis

fMRI (Functional Magnetic Resonance Imaging)

A type of noninvasive imaging study that allows the observer to visualize the areas of the brain that are functioning after exposure to a particular brain activity.

PART THREE

Risk, Prevention, and Epidemiology

What risk factors contribute to people smoking?

Does my risk for a specific illness related to smoking change after I quit smoking?

How do I know if my child will become a smoker?

More . . .

RISK

34. If I am addicted to tobacco, will I be predisposed to other addictions?

Smokers are far more likely to develop an addiction to tobacco and far less likely to successfully quit than people who use other addictive drugs. It is harder to break a smoking addiction than a heroin addiction. And while the majority of smokers are not addicted to other drugs, the majority of drug and alcohol addicts are also addicted to smoking. It appears that all addictions—whether they are street drugs, alcohol, tobacco, or certain behaviors such as gambling, sex, or even shopping—are mediated at some level via the brain's reward system and its principal neurotransmitter, dopamine (see Question 7). We know this from a variety of sources both direct and indirect. Laboratory research has found an overlap between the effects of nicotine and opiates on dopamine signaling. Additionally, certain drugs known as dopamine agonists prescribed for Parkinson's disease have unusual side effects, including an increase in sexual behavior, gambling, and shopping. The dopamine reuptake inhibitor **bupropion**, which increases the amount of dopamine in the brain, has aided patients in smoking cessation. Nicotine and alcohol also influence the body's internal opiate system, known collectively as endorphins, which cause **analgesia** and euphoria, which also affects the dopamine system. One of three medications approved for the treatment of alcoholism is naltrexone, which blocks the opiate receptors and thereby reduces craving for alcohol. Finally, brain imaging studies have demonstrated that various drugs of abuse activate the same areas of the brain in addition to their own individual actions. These overlapping areas are pathways regarded to be part of the brain's reward system.

All in all, the susceptibility to develop any addiction is general. But the odds of becoming addicted vary not only with one's own genetic susceptibility but also with the type of drug one is using, because some drugs are more prone to cause

Bupropion

Generic name for the drugs Wellbutrin, marketed as an antidepressant, and Zyban, marketed as a smoking cessation medication.

Analgesia

A type of drug that relieves pain. Analgesics include nonsteroidal anti-inflammatory (NSAIDs) agents such as aspirin and opiates such as morphine.

addiction than others. Given that nicotine has a greater addictive potential than other drugs, more people will become addicted to it, including those who are not generally susceptible to addiction. Individuals who are more highly susceptible to addiction will very quickly become addicted to nicotine along with a variety of other drugs they might use on a regular basis. Thus, becoming addicted to tobacco does not necessarily predict that one is more susceptible to other addictions. What does predict susceptibility, however, is the speed with which one becomes addicted, and this is often determined by the age of first use and the age when one begins to use regularly. Early use of tobacco and early heavy use of tobacco especially, is a strong predictor for the susceptibility of becoming addicted to other drugs (see Question 16).

35. What risk factors contribute to people smoking?

Risk factors are the characteristics that increase the chances of developing a disease or disorder. Epidemiology is the study of disease or disorder rates in large populations, and the various circumstances both biologically and environmentally that are common among individuals who develop a particular disease or disorder under study. It is through these studies that risk factors for a particular condition are discovered. Some risk factors are modifiable, which means the individual can lower his or her risk for developing a particular condition by making changes in his or her life, such as modifying diet, activity, or exposure. Some risk factors are non-modifiable, which means that the individual has no ability to lower or modify the risk, such as gender or other heritable traits.

It appears that teens become addicted more quickly because of developmental and biological factors.

The following is a list of risk factors associated with the development of nicotine dependency:

- *Age:* It appears that teens become addicted more quickly because of developmental and biological factors.
- *Gender:* A higher percentage of teen smokers are males. More white females smoke than other ethnic groups.

Adult males were more likely to smoke, but that has changed now that more women are joining the workforce and are exposed to other smokers. Females have more difficulty quitting than males.

- *Ethnicity:* Higher rates of smoking are found among Caucasians and Native Americans; lower rates of smoking are found among African Americans, Latino Americans, and Asian Americans.

- *Geographical area in the United States:* Higher rates of smoking are found in the southern tobacco-growing states and the Midwest as well as Nevada; the lowest rates of tobacco use are in the West, namely Utah (The Mormon religion forbids smoking).

- *Mental illness*: A higher percentage of the mentally ill are heavy smokers.

- *Children and adolescents with neuropsychiatric disorders:* Higher rates of smoking are seen in young people diagnosed with attention deficit hyperactivity disorder (**ADHD**) and conduct disorders.

- *Alcoholism:* There is a strong association between the two addictions. If you attend an Alcoholics Anonymous meeting, most likely you will find yourself in a smoke-filled room.

- *Poor education or lower socio-economic class*: Today, there are more smokers among the poor and uneducated than among the middle class, the wealthy, and the well-educated.

- *Living in a developing country:* Smoking rates are higher in the developing nations.

- *Parental and peer smoking*: Role modeling is a powerful learning tool. Rates of smoking increase in families where the parents smoke. An even stronger influence is the peer group. Teens are far more likely to smoke if their teenage peers smoke than if their parents smoke.

Attention Deficit Hyperactivity Disorder (ADHD)

A persistent pattern of inattention and/or hyperactivity, impulsivity that is seen more frequently in children with ADHD than in children at comparable developmental levels.

36. What are the risks of secondhand or environmental smoke?

In 1991, the Environmental Protection Agency (EPA) reported that 20% of lung cancers diagnosed among nonsmokers were due to exposure to environmental tobacco smoke, making the risk of developing a smoking-related disease 1:1000, higher than all chemically related environments regulated by the EPA. Today, secondhand smoke is thought to contribute to about 3400 lung cancer deaths and 23,000 to 70,000 cardiovascular deaths in U.S. nonsmokers annually. It is especially harmful to young children and is thought to be responsible for between 150,000 and 300,000 respiratory tract infections in children under 18 months of age, resulting in between 7500 and 15,000 hospitalizations annually. It is thought to be one of the causes of sudden infant death syndrome (SIDS). The most recent *Surgeon General's Report* concluded that even brief exposures to secondhand smoke can cause blood **platelets** to become stickier, damage the lining of blood vessels, decrease coronary artery blood flow, and increase the risk of an acute heart attack.

Following this report, there has been progress in improving the number of workplaces that are smoke-free. National trends for smoke-free environments have continued to improve from 46.3% in the years 1992–1993 to 70.9% in 2001–2002.

37. Does my risk for a specific illness related to smoking change after I quit smoking?

If you stop smoking, the benefits to your health and longevity are great. Becoming smoke free has health benefits no matter how long you have smoked. The body starts repairing itself almost immediately after smoking cessation, but some organs may not be able to recover completely, depending upon the length of time you have smoked.

Platelets

(Also known as thrombocytes.) A type of blood cell involved in the cellular mechanisms of the formation of blood clots. Low levels or dysfunction predisposes for bleeding, while high levels, although usually asymptomatic, may increase the risk of the development of a thrombus.

In general, the excess risk among former smokers drops substantially in the first two to three years. Thereafter, the rate of decline decreases so that it takes up to 10 years for former smokers to reach the same risk level as that of persons who have never smoked. The slow decline in all morbidity and mortality due to coronary heart disease is related to reversal of some atherogenic effects of smoking. The risk of myocardial infarction diminishes by almost one-third after the first year of smoking cessation and reaches the level of persons who have never smoked by the third or fourth year. The rapid decline in heart attack (myocardial infarction) risk is thought to be due to a rapid reversal of hypercoagulability induced by smoking. The risk of sudden death due to all cardiovascular events takes longer to be reduced to nonsmokers' levels, anywhere from 5 to 15 years.

38. What are my chances of recovery from smoking-related diseases such as cardiac disease, lung cancer, chronic pulmonary disease (including emphysema), and stroke?

It is important to remember that all of these diseases can occur independently of whether or not someone smokes. These diseases are age related, and diet, activity, and exposure to other environmental toxins can contribute to their development. Never having smoked is no guarantee one will avoid these diseases. Therefore, quitting smoking is no guarantee of avoiding them either. Smoking merely increases the risk and accelerates the course of the disease once someone has developed it. With that in mind, quitting smoking certainly lowers one's risk and slows down the progress of disease. So the real issue is whether or not quitting lowers the risk back to nonsmokers' levels.

Cardiovascular Diseases: These are diseases of the heart or blood vessels (arteries and veins). Heart disease kills more Americans than cancer. A six-year follow-up study of people older than 55 years, who were smokers, found that the death rate was significantly higher among smokers who continued to smoke than among those who had quit. It takes anywhere between 5 and 15 years after one quits smoking to lower one's risk back to that of a nonsmoker.

Lung Cancer: Smoking cessation reduces lung cancer risk by 30% to 50% 10 years after quitting. The risk that you will develop lung cancer decreases with further years of abstinence. The risk of lung cancer is always a possibility though when compared to someone who has never smoked. For example, approximately 50% of all lung cancers are diagnosed in ex-smokers.

Chronic Obstructive Pulmonary Disease, Including Emphysema: Chronic obstructive pulmonary disease (COPD) is a term for a group of lung conditions that restrict airflow, making breathing difficult. The conditions include:

- Emphysema: breathlessness caused by damage to the air sacs (alveoli) causing them to become less elastic.
- Chronic bronchitis: coughing with a lot of mucus that continues for at least three months.

Smoking is the most common cause of COPD and is responsible for 80% of cases. Approximately 90% of 1 pack/day smokers have some emphysema on postmortem examination, while more than 90% of nonsmokers have little or no emphysema on postmortem examination. COPD typically occurs after the age of 40, when lung function starts to decline anyway.

In smokers, the rate of decline in lung function can be three times the rate of nonsmokers. As the condition progresses, severe breathing problems can require hospital care. The final stage is death from slow suffocation, which is a progressive loss of the ability to oxygenate the body. The rate of decline may or may not revert to that of a nonsmoker. If lung damage has occurred due to smoking, the damage may never be completely repaired. This means that the lung function will still be diminished compared to someone who has never smoked.

Stroke: A stroke occurs when there is a rapid loss of brain function because of a disturbance in the blood vessels that carry blood to the brain. Strokes can be thought of as brain attacks in the same manner that people suffer heart attacks. The mechanism is the same, except the atherosclerotic buildup is located in the major arteries supplying blood to the brain as opposed to the heart. As a result, the risk of stroke follows the same general pattern as the risk of coronary artery disease.

Within a few years after quitting smoking, the risk of having a stroke decreases. The risk of stroke is highest in smokers under age 55 and decreases with age. There is also a dose-response effect between the number of cigarettes smoked and risk of stroke. Researchers have found strong correlations between smoking and thrombotic stroke (slow decrease in blood supply), embolic stroke (sudden release of a blood clot), and subarachnoid hemorrhage (blood leaking from the vessels and pooling in the brain). The relative risk of subarachnoid hemorrhage was significantly higher than that of thrombotic stroke.

39. If I don't inhale will I have less of a chance of getting a disease, such as lung cancer?

It is important to remember that there both direct and indirect risks from smoking, whether or not one inhales. You are still exposing your body to tar and nicotine. While not inhaling reduces the direct exposure of tar and nicotine to the lungs, it does not eliminate exposure. Smokers who do not inhale are still breathing secondhand smoke and continue to be at risk for lung cancer. Additionally, the carcinogenic effects of tar and nicotine are still absorbed by the body, and therefore the risk of a variety of cancers, such as bladder cancer and pancreatic cancer, remains unchanged. While the direct toxicity of tar and nicotine is reduced to the lungs, it continues to have direct toxic effects to the mouth, gums, teeth, tongue, nasal linings, and esophagus. Pipe and cigar smokers, who often do not inhale, are at an increased risk for lip, mouth, tongue, and

While not inhaling reduces the direct exposure of tar and nicotine to the lungs, it does not eliminate exposure.

some other cancers. Even limited smoking, such as one or two cigarettes per day, or inhaling three to five grams of tobacco per day (environmental smoke) puts your health at risk.

PREVENTION

40. What is the "Great American Smoke Out"?

"The Great American Smoke Out" is an annual event sponsored by The American Cancer Society. On November 18, 1976, the California Division of the American Cancer Society successfully prompted nearly one million smokers to quit smoking for a day. That event marked the first "Great American Smoke Out," which has now become a yearly nationwide event.

"The Great American Smoke Out" has helped to bring about dramatic changes in Americans' attitudes about smoking. Changing attitudes have paved the way for changes in organizations and institutions so that fewer Americans are exposed to secondhand smoke than ever before, and it has led the way to the development of community programs that focus on prevention and smoking cessation.

41. What anti-tobacco education is being done in the schools? How effective are programs such as DARE?

DARE (Drug Abuse Resistance Education) is an international program for school age children and teens to prevent the use of tobacco and illegal drugs, membership in gangs, and violence. It is a collaborative effort by law enforcement, educators, parents, and community leaders. DARE was founded in 1983 by the Los Angeles Police Department. It promoted the presence of police in the classroom as the most appropriate teachers for school children to learn that drugs and violence kill.

The goals of the program are to foster resiliency in young people, to improve their capacity to make healthy decisions, and to enhance independent growth and self-reliance. Students learn to substitute healthy activities and to avoid participating in risky behaviors, such as drug abuse, violence, and other destructive behaviors.

Police officers undergo 80 hours of special training in child development, classroom management, teaching techniques, and communication skills. The prevention program is comprehensive and age appropriate.

The curriculum for elementary students includes:

- Tobacco smoking and advertising
- Drug abuse
- Inhalants
- Alcohol consumption
- Health and healthy lifestyles
- Peer pressure in a social network

The high school curriculum is a reinforcement of the information provided at the primary level and adds how to:

- Act in one's own best interest when facing high-risk, low-gain choices.
- Resist peer pressure and other influences in making personal choices.

Funding comes from multiple sources: The Department of Education, The Department of Justice and The U.S. Drug Enforcement Administration, The U.S. Office of Justice and Delinquency Prevention, corporations, private foundations, individual contributions, state legislatures, local school districts, religious organizations, and local businesses, as well as youth organizations. Funding also may come from a State's Master Settlement payments.

Results Regarding the Effectiveness of These Programs Conflict

School-Based Programs are Effective: More than 20 studies conducted from around the country have documented that 93% of the children and young people who are DARE graduates have never tried drugs, 75% have never tried tobacco products, and 90% of the graduates stated that they learned to resist the temptation to try drugs and learned to deal effectively with peer pressure. In another study, the results showed that the use of illicit drugs among teens declined from 11.6% in 2002 to 8.8% in 2006. The reduced percentage of teens using marijuana was particularly pronounced.

School-Based Programs are Ineffective: DARE has become so controversial that many school districts have discontinued the program or substituted other programs for DARE. The Hutchinson Smoking Prevention Project conducted a long-term evaluation study of smoking prevention programs in Washington State school districts. It was one of the most rigorous studies conducted on smoking prevention in the schools. The study spanned 10 years across grades 3 to 12. The study concluded that the DARE school smoking prevention programs do not work, especially when the curriculum does not take into consideration family and community cultural norms.

The following are a few of the other criticisms:

- DARE is ineffective and may have the opposite effect, promoting drug use.
- DARE is ineffective in reducing violence.
- DARE suppresses unfavorable research, rejects scientific evidence, and questions critics' integrity.
- DARE misinforms, teaching that all drugs are equally dangerous.
- DARE, by using policemen, the symbol of authority, may negatively influence a student to be against the police.

- DARE undermines the family. Part of the program has a lesson entitled, "The Three R's: Recognize, Resist, Report," which encourages children to report if they find drugs in their homes.
- DARE is a waste of time and money and should be replaced by a more effective program.

Although the outcomes of studies conflict, there is evidence that school-based programs are effective for some children and teens. The Surgeon General's 1994 *Report* found that after years of research on a wide variety of school-based programs, most of them demonstrated success in reducing tobacco use.

Two *Morbidity and Mortality Weekly Reports* (*MMWR*) showed that comprehensive school-based programs, combined with community and media-based activities were effective in preventing or postponing the onset of smoking in 20% to 40% of U.S. adolescents. The second report quoted recommendations from the National Cancer Institute advisory panel, which stated that prevention programs should include the following: the social and short-term physiological consequences of tobacco use; training students in refusal skills; involvement of parents, teachers, and peers in smoking-prevention activities; and reflection of the needs of each community, so that the program is culturally sensitive.

Recommendations from the Institute of Medicine (IOM) are that school-based programs should be comprehensive, be integrated into school health programs, be sequential across grade levels, use many different strategies, activities, and services, and be designed to promote physical, emotional, and social health, as well as providing prevention. The IOM recommended that the anti-smoking program should be designed by an interdisciplinary team of teachers and that the team should be accountable to the community. The overall conclusion from the conflicting studies is that there is no one "best program" that fits all communities. Programs should be designed locally in collaboration with all of the community's stakeholders.

42. What are the other prevention programs for children?

The No Tobacco Use Program (TNT Program). Muskegon County, Michigan developed its own tobacco prevention program, called the *TNT Program*. Upon completion of the program, the prevalence of tobacco use among teens declined.

The American Stop Smoking Intervention (ASSIST). The American Cancer Society partnered with the National Cancer Institute and local health departments to launch the *ASSIST* program in a number of communities. It is a multimodal approach to prevention and smoking cessation. The interventions include the media to increase pro-tobacco-control coverage, strengthening indoor clean air laws, and reducing youth access to tobacco.

ASPIRE. ASPIRE is another smoking prevention school-based program. It includes a CD-ROM animation-based curriculum developed at the University of Texas Science Center at Houston. It is an interactive school curriculum with animation and video game elements, targeted to students in the 10th to 12th grades. The topical outline includes:

- The short- and long-term effects of smoking
- Social issues
- The addictive nature of smoking
- Tobacco advertising
- Society's move from smoking as an acceptable activity to now when it is unacceptable
- Financial issues

The Youth Tobacco Prevention Policies and Programs in Schools and Communities, developed by The Department of Health and Human Services (DHHS). DHHS developed a curriculum for Tobacco Prevention in the public schools. They advised the use of peer educators and parents to teach children about the effects of smoking. DHHS suggested that the consequences of smoking on school grounds should be clearly communicated to all students, should involve both school officials and law enforcement, and should be consistently applied. Prevention programs should be across grade levels and should include health and social issues, resistance skills, and the influence of advertising on people's choices. Besides classroom teaching, they recommended the establishment of a peer-to-peer mentoring program to support abstinence. Other suggestions are to supplement classroom education using the Internet and other media sources. The Internet has great appeal to young people because it provides an environment that can be graphically appealing, anonymous, and non-judgmental. It can also provide ongoing support.

Other smoking cessation programs may not be exactly like the DARE program but have similar components. Many schools have integrated tobacco and drug prevention into their health courses rather than having a stand-alone program. Communities and schools have joined forces to develop programs that use a multimodal approach, are culturally sensitive, and meet the needs of their population.

43. How old should my child be before I talk to him or her about smoking?

The Center for Disease Control and Prevention (CDC) recommends that parents start a dialogue with their children about the use of tobacco by ages 5 or 6. Continue talking to your children through high school. If you wait until they are preteens, it may be too late. Many kids start using tobacco by age 11 years and many are addicted by age 14. Parents, grandparents, coaches, teachers, and other adults should keep communication ongoing and openly discuss tobacco and other drugs. Introduce the subject of smoking when a child is very young in simple language according to the child's developmental age and in terms that the child can understand.

If you wait until they are preteens, it may be too late.

44. How do I talk to my child about smoking?

The following guidelines will help you communicate with your child.

- Clearly state your own values.

- Focus on the immediate short-term consequences, such as bad breath, smelly clothes, yellow teeth, and poor performance in sports. Only discuss long-term consequences with teens, who understand the concept of links between tobacco use and disease and death.

- Be a good role model. Actions speak louder than words. Kids do what you do and not what you say. If you do smoke, then do not smoke in front of your children and don't leave cigarettes where they can be easily reached. If a toddler eats cigarettes, it can be fatal. The best thing you can do for your child is to quit. Tell your children the reasons why you do not want them to smoke. Be honest. Share your mistakes. If you do smoke, tell them about your own struggles with addiction. Tell why you wish you had never started. Know that you may be effective in preventing your child from smoking, if you do quit. One-third of the children whose parents quit smoking are less likely to smoke.

- Help children to cope with life's stressors. Listen, empathize, be supportive, and allow them to express their feelings. "*Feelings are OK.*" Build their self-esteem and self-confidence.

- Discuss problems and teach problem-solving skills. Allow them to make some of their own decisions that are age appropriate.

- Make household rules clear. Be consistent. Spell out the consequences for breaking the rules and do not hesitate to enforce them when necessary.

- Monitor the TV programs they watch, movies your child attends, the magazines they read, computer games they play, and their use of the Internet. Talk about how advertisers glamorize smoking and drinking and that the information found in advertisements gives a false impression.

- Participate in family dinners, family rituals, bedtime rituals, and family games and outings. Family togetherness is a great preventative strategy.

Teach your children how to cope with peer pressure. Most of the difficulties that children have to face are the social pressures from other kids. Practice with your child and/or role-play examples of how to handle peer pressure.

Parents are the most important resource in preventing teen substance abuse, including smoking.

45. How do I know if my child will become a smoker?

Studies demonstrate that the two most important predictors determining your child's risk of becoming a smoker are access to cigarettes and friends who smoke. The following is a quiz to assess the risk of your child becoming a smoker.

- *Does your child hang around with other kids who smoke cigarettes?*
  The smoking rate among kids who have three or more friends who smoke is 10 times higher than the rate among kids whose friends are smoke-free.

- *Do you or your spouse smoke?*
  Studies have shown that kids whose parents are smokers are at least twice as likely to smoke.

- *Do your child's siblings smoke?*
  Having an older brother or sister who smokes triples the odds that a younger sibling will smoke.

- *Is your child having trouble in school?*
Smoking is linked to poor academic achievement.

- *Does your child have a lot of unsupervised time after school?*
Children who engage in structured after-school programs, such as clubs or sports, have a lower risk of smoking. Be involved in what your children are doing, and know the children and families with whom your children are involved.

- *Is your child depressed?*
Several studies have linked cigarette smoking with symptoms of depression among adolescents.

- *Is your child an adolescent?*
Children ages 11 to 15 in grades 6 to 10 are most vulnerable to peer influences and are most likely to try their first cigarette. If a friend or relative has died from a tobacco-related illness, talk to your teenage son or daughter about this person's death.

46. Should I enroll my child in a prevention program?

School-based programs will support your conversations with your child about smoking, thus reinforcing the no smoking rule in your household. If your school does not have a tobacco prevention program, find a program for your child in your local area. Then suggest through the Parent Teachers Association (PTA) that your school develop one. The information found in these questions should give you ideas about designing a program for your school and community. Not only will your child benefit from attending a prevention program, but if you are smoker, you will benefit, too.

47. My spouse is a heavy smoker who refuses to get help to quit. What should I do?

There is not much you can do until he or she is ready to quit. Many smokers have tried to quit but have not been successful. Consequently, they have "given up." Others remember the discomforts of the withdrawal symptoms and would rather not have to go through that experience again. Other people freely admit that they love to smoke and do not want to give it up. Different personalities and different experiences contribute to different attitudes toward smoking.

Many smokers do not realize that new ways are available to assist smokers to quit, which may decrease the negative experiences of withdrawal. If the smoker is willing to think about the possibility of quitting, a spouse can help by collecting information about smoking cessation programs and provide his or her loved one with information about the opportunities for quitting.

A "Change Model," or the "Trans-Theoretical Model" is a process model that identifies stages that a smoker must traverse in order to achieve abstinence. The stages are:

- **Pre-contemplation:** The person is aware that he or she has a problem but has not seriously thought about making a change.
- **Contemplation:** The person begins to see that the behavior is a problem and seriously considers making a change but remains ambivalent about doing so.
- **Preparation:** The person has decided to make a change and has a specific plan to do so in the near future.
- **Action:** The person implements an action plan and begins to make the desired changes.
- **Maintenance:** The person has made the desired change and works to avoid relapsing into the original behavior (smoking).
- **Termination:** The person is safely through the process, experiences zero temptation, and has the ability to resist any temptation 100% of the time.

If a spouse understands these phases, he or she can help a loved one along the pathway to abstinence. During the pre-contemplation and contemplation stages, if the loved one is open to discussion, the spouse can provide information, and also they can talk about a future plan to quit and what the spouse can do to help the smoker quit. Together they can identify a "quit" date. The spouse can provide empathy and support during the next two phases, preparation and action. The nonsmoker spouse may have to overlook the irritability that the smoker is feeling that may lead to some negative behaviors. The "blues" also may contribute to behavior changes. The negatives should be ignored and the positives should be supported. The spouse can help with the maintenance phase by ensuring that the couple's social life takes place only in smoke-free environments and that they socialize solely with nonsmokers. The spouse should constantly offer support during the maintenance and termination stages as well as throughout the withdrawal process. A supportive, loving relationship can go a long way to helping the smoker along the path to a healthy lifestyle.

Joseph's comment:

For many years, I dabbled in trying to quit here and there with little success. Even with the physical ramifications of smoking starting to affect my body, I seemed to have no success. No matter how many people tried to help and encourage me from the outside, I truly don't think I could get on the journey to quitting until I hit my own personal bottom. I tried "smoking cessations" once before, with no luck. Like the old saying goes, "If at first you don't succeed, try, try, again." My second time around, when it came up to the quit date, I put the cigarette down, using the "patch" as an aid, and made it through the first 24 hours. I was so filled with hope that I tried for another day and succeeded. At that point, I felt I was in a "zone." I stopped looking at it as quitting forever and just not smoking one day at a time.

EPIDEMIOLOGY

48. *What is* Healthy People 2010*? Is smoking cessation included in its national goals?*

The Department of Health and Human Services (DHHS) has been setting national objectives for Americans' health since the 1980s when it first published *Health Objectives for the Nation*. Subsequently, it published *Healthy People 2000* and recently *Healthy People 2010*. DHHS is responsible for overseeing the nation's health. Their goals have been established to improve the health status of the U.S. population as well as the availability and quality of health services so the life span of Americans can be extended. DHHS encourages the establishment of prevention programs, including smoking cessation, and monitors the national health status and the achievement of the goals set in the *Healthy People 2000* and *2010* reports. Every ten years, a *Healthy People* report that addresses the national public health trends is presented to the Secretary of DHHS, the President, and the U.S. Congress. The report also includes goals on prevention and strategies to be achieved over the next 10-year period. Both *Healthy People 2000* and *2010* have two overarching goals: to increase the quality of health care during each American's lifetime and to eliminate health disparities. Ten indicators are used to measure the nation's health. Each of the indicators reflects a major health concern. The health indicators are listed as follows:

1. Physical activity
2. Overweight and obesity
3. Tobacco use
4. Substance abuse
5. Responsible sexual behavior
6. Mental health
7. Injury and violence
8. Environmental quality
9. Immunization
10. Access to health care

The indicators 3, 4, and 8 are factors involving tobacco use and addiction. Health indicators are selected based on the ability to motivate the public to act, the availability of the data to measure progress, and the importance of the indicator to the overall health of Americans. The selection process is done by consensus. The authors of the document are from both the private and public sectors of communities across the country. The report is the outcome of a shared vision about improving the health of the nation, preventing disease, and improving the quality of life of all citizens.

The *Healthy People* reports are used by many organizations, communities, and policy-makers to measure, compare, and improve the health status of local communities. Information for specific health issues is also developed and distributed to special populations, such as gays and lesbians, people with disabilities, rural health populations, women's health organizations, and healthcare professionals who work with special populations. *Healthy People 2010* provides a framework for health advocates to develop strategies to improve access to quality health care. Many public health officials consider tobacco-related diseases as the most critical healthcare concern, particularly because these diseases are easily preventable through public education, legislation, and the development of prevention and cessation programs.

49. What are the rights of smokers and nonsmokers?

Smokers' organizations throughout the United States have developed to combat what they perceive has been a systematic effort to deprive them of their rights. The two main organizations are the American Smokers Alliance and the National Smokers Alliance. Other smokers' rights groups with international membership include Freedom Organization for the Right to Enjoy Smoking Tobacco (FOREST) and Fight Ordinances and Restrictions to Control and Eliminate Smoking (FORCES). Controversy has surrounded these organizations due to their link with tobacco companies.

Risk, Prevention, and Epidemiology

Smoker's Rights

The following are the Smokers' Bill of Rights:

As a smoker, I am entitled to certain inalienable rights, among them:

- The right to the pursuit of happiness
- The right to choose to smoke
- The right to enjoy a traditional American custom
- The right to be treated courteously
- The right to accommodation in the workplace
- The right to accommodation in public places
- The right to unrestricted access to commercial information about products
- The right to purchase products without excessive taxation
- The right to freedom from unnecessary government intrusion

If you do a Google search using "smokers' rights" as keywords, the R.J. Reynolds Tobacco Company comes up at the top of the list. In order to better understand the perspective of the tobacco company's positions regarding smokers' rights and the sale of cigarettes, you may visit their Web site. Below is a short excerpt that gives an example of their guiding principles and beliefs:

Guiding Principles and Beliefs

TOBACCO USE & HEALTH

- Nicotine in tobacco products is addictive but is not considered a significant threat to health.
- No tobacco product has been shown to be safe.
- An individual's level of risk for serious disease is significantly affected by the type of tobacco product used as well as the manner and frequency of use.

TOBACCO REGULATION

- Tobacco products should be regulated in a reasonable and consistent manner, and they should remain legal and consumer-acceptable. The prohibition, in any form, of tobacco products is neither practical nor desirable.

- Smoking restrictions should exempt adult venues such as bars and taverns.

HARM REDUCTION

- Decreasing the health risks and harm directly associated with the use of tobacco products is in everyone's best interest.

- Adult tobacco consumers should have access to a range of tobacco, nicotine and cessation products and should be given information in order to make an informed choice on the relative risks of each product.

Nonsmoker's Rights

Organizations like the Group Against Smoking and Pollution (GASP), founded in 1971, developed anti-smoking chapters throughout the country to limit smoking in public areas, including restaurants, airplanes, trains, and buses. The organization developed a Bill of Rights for Nonsmokers. It focused attention on environmental smoke. By the 1990s, anti-smoking groups and public health advocates had effectively influenced state legislators to limit public use of tobacco products. By then, consumers no longer tolerated even low risks to health from secondary smoke. The following is the Bill of Rights for Nonsmokers.

I have the right to:

- Be smoke-free in any situation

- Review my list of reasons to stop smoking frequently, particularly before any social gathering

- Ask others not to smoke in my home, office, or car

- Sit in nonsmoking sections

- Support legislation to protect nonsmokers from the dangers of passive smoking in public places

50. What are the current trends in quitting smoking?

The number of smokers in the United States is declining, as public awareness regarding the dangers of smoking have become more widely accepted and more local communities are banning smoking in public places. Among Americans, smoking rates shrunk by nearly half in three decades (from the mid-1960s to mid-1990s), falling to 23% of adults by 1997. However, worldwide, especially in poor countries, the number of smokers is growing. In the developing world, tobacco consumption is rising by 3.4% per year. In the developing world, concerns about the use of tobacco are not considered as important as concerns about adequate nutrition, safe drinking water, and communicable diseases.

51. What is the prevalence of tobacco use?

Prevalence refers to the current number of people suffering from a particular illness or engaged in a particular activity relative to the population at large over a specified period of time. *Point prevalence* refers to a defined point in time (such as January 1, 2009) while *period prevalence* refers to a defined period in time (such as January 1, 2008 through January 1, 2009). It is defined in terms of the ratio of people with a condition compared to the total population.

Today one out of every five adults smokes regularly. A 2007 *Time* magazine article on the "Science of Addiction" reported that there are 71.5 million tobacco users in the United States, of whom 23.4% are men and 18.5% are women. Among cigarette smokers, the lowest rate of smokers live in the western section of the country and the highest live in the Midwest and the southeast tobacco-producing states. The proportion of smokers in the adult population has fallen from a high of 46% in 1950 to 21% in 2004. The World Health Organization in 2003 estimated that there were 1.3 billion smokers worldwide. The numbers may vary from source to source, but all of the data point to a worldwide epidemic of pandemic proportions (**Table 7**).

Table 7   Smoking Prevalence

Region	Percent of Smokers	
	Men	Women
Africa	29	4
United States	35	22
Eastern Mediterranean	35	4
Europe	46	26
Southeast Asia	44	4
Western Pacific	60	8

Source: 2000, World Health Organization estimates.

The numbers are expected to reach 7 billion by 2025. The growth will be among people living in poor developing countries and the uneducated.

52. What are the mortality rates from smoking in the United States? Worldwide?

Mortality rates are the rates of deaths in a population during a given time and in a given place. Smoking kills over 435,000 U.S. citizens each year. More Americans die each year from tobacco than from fires, car accidents, illegal drugs, murders, and AIDS combined. Tobacco kills more people in two days than crack and cocaine kill in a year. More than 50,000 Americans die from secondhand smoke, according to the Centers for Disease Control and Prevention (CDC). Sixteen million people lost their lives because of an addiction to nicotine between 1950 and 2000. These numbers add up to a thousand American deaths each day from smoking cigarettes. Most of the deaths occur to people between the ages of 35 and 69 years. Nearly five million people died from smoking worldwide in 2000, and smoking killed nearly as many people in developing countries as in developed countries. The World Health Organization (WHO) estimates that tobacco kills a person every 10 seconds worldwide and, at the current growth rate for both the general population and number of smokers, the death rate from smoking may exceed 10 million a year in 30 years.

Risk, Prevention, and Epidemiology

PART FOUR

Treatment

What is the current trend in smoking cessation treatment?

How successful are people who quit on their own?

What can I do to avoid "triggers"?

More . . .

53. How successful will I be at quitting smoking?

Epidemiologic data report that 70% of the 45 million smokers in the United States today want to quit, and approximately 44% try to quit each year. The vast majority of these attempts are without support and are unsuccessful. Only 4% to 7% will actually succeed. These statistics may discourage both smokers and clinicians because the majority of smokers struggle through multiple periods of abstinence and relapse.

The introduction of numerous effective treatments in the past 15 to 20 years now gives the clinician and patient many additional options over the long haul.

Because of the chronic, relapsing nature of tobacco dependency, the most effective way to understand and treat it is by recognizing it as a chronic disease. By approaching it as a chronic disease, clinicians will better accept its relapsing nature and the requirement for ongoing, long-term care, which includes continued patient education, counseling, and advice over time. These strategies are similar to the way you would approach other chronic diseases such as diabetes, hypertension, or asthma. The introduction of numerous effective treatments in the past 15 to 20 years now gives the clinician and patient many additional options over the long haul. Clinicians should provide tobacco-dependent patients with brief advice, counseling, and appropriate medication. Assessing and treating tobacco use as a chronic disease generally leads to greater patient satisfaction and improved success at eventually quitting.

Joseph's comment:

Quite honestly, while I was smoking, I did not think I could be successful. Something inside me kept making me try different techniques. It wasn't until I put the cigarette down for a few 24 hour periods that I really started to believe I could be successful, and there was hope for me becoming a nonsmoker.

54. What is the current trend in smoking cessation treatment?

In 2008, the U.S. Department of Health and Human Services (DHHS) published an update of clinical practice guidelines entitled *Treating Tobacco Use and Dependence*. It provided 10 key recommendations, which are listed here. These practice guidelines are available online for free at http://www.surgeongeneral .gov/tobacco/.

The overarching goal of these recommendations is that clinicians strongly recommend the use of effective tobacco dependence counseling and medication treatments to their patients who use tobacco, and that health systems, insurers, and purchasers assist clinicians in making such effective treatments available.

Ten Key Guideline Recommendations

1. Tobacco dependence is a chronic disease that often requires repeated intervention and multiple attempts to quit. Effective treatments exist, however, that can significantly increase rates of long-term abstinence.

2. It is essential that clinicians and healthcare delivery systems consistently identify and document tobacco use status and treat every tobacco user seen in a healthcare setting.

3. Tobacco dependence treatments are effective across a broad range of populations. Clinicians should encourage every patient willing to make a quit attempt to use the counseling treatments and medications recommended in this Guideline.

4. Brief tobacco dependence treatment is effective. Clinicians should offer every patient who uses tobacco at least the brief treatments shown to be effective.

5. Individual, group, and telephone counseling are effective, and their effectiveness increases with treatment intensity. Two components of counseling are especially effective, and clinicians should use these when counseling patients making a quit attempt:

   • Practical counseling (problem solving and skills training)

   • Social support delivered as part of treatment

6. Numerous effective medications are available for tobacco dependence, and clinicians should encourage their use by all patients attempting to quit smoking. Clinicians also should encourage their use by all patient populations attempting to quit for whom there is insufficient evidence of effectiveness (that is, pregnant women, smokeless tobacco users, light smokers, and adolescents). Seven first-line medications (5 nicotine and 2 non-nicotine) reliably increase long-term smoking abstinence rates:

   • Bupropion SR (Zyban or Wellbutrin)

   • Nicotine gum

   • Nicotine inhaler

   • Nicotine lozenge

   • Nicotine nasal spray

   • Nicotine patch

   • Varenicline (Chantix)

   Clinicians also should consider the use of certain combinations of medications identified as effective in this Guideline.

7. Counseling and medication are effective when used by themselves for treating tobacco dependence. The combination of counseling and medication, however, is more effective than either therapy alone. Thus, clinicians should encourage all individuals making a quit attempt to use both counseling and medication.

8. Telephone "quitline" counseling is effective with diverse populations and has a broad reach. Therefore, both clinicians and healthcare delivery systems should ensure patient access to quitlines and promote quitline use.

9. If a tobacco user currently is unwilling to make a quit attempt, clinicians should use the motivational treatments shown to be effective in increasing future quit attempts.

10. Tobacco dependence treatments are both clinically effective and highly cost-effective relative to interventions for other clinical disorders. Providing coverage for these treatments increases quit rates. Insurers and purchasers should ensure that all insurance plans include the counseling and medication identified as effective in this Guideline as covered benefits.

In addition to the 10 key recommendations, the Guideline also cites "The Five A's" as a model for treating alcohol use and dependence. They are listed here:

The Five A's Model for Treating Tobacco Use and Dependence

1. Ask about tobacco use. Identify and document tobacco use status for every patient at every visit.

2. Advise to quit. In a clear, strong, and personalized manner, urge every tobacco user to quit.

3. Assess willingness to make a quit attempt. Is the tobacco user willing to make a quit attempt at this time?

4. Assist in quit attempt. For the patient willing to make a quit attempt, offer medication and provide or refer for counseling or additional treatment to help the patient quit. For patients unwilling to quit at the time, provide interventions designed to increase future quit attempts.

5. Arrange follow-up. For the patient willing to make a quit attempt, arrange for follow-up contacts, beginning within the first week after the quit date. For patients unwilling to make a quit attempt at the time, address tobacco dependence and willingness to quit at the next clinic visit.

Lisa's comment:

I feel, after trying various processes to quit in the past, that it was having all my "forces" lined up behind me. In retrospect, I see that I had so many layers of support that mentally, I was thinking if one thing didn't work, I had another thing to fall back on; there was one layer after another. I utilized every "tool" available to me: my GP, a therapist, a cessation program, medication (Zyban, at that time), nicotine supplements (patch and gum), a self-hypnosis tape, a quiz to determine what kind of smoker I was, homework, acupressure, and a support group. I, who smoked two and a half packs a day for 30 years, have successfully lived my life entirely smoke-free now for 6 years. Before the combination of tools listed, I had only managed to struggle to 14 days before falling apart and smoking again.

55. What are the qualifications of professionals who run smoking cessation groups?

Qualifications of those who run smoking cessation groups vary. People who run smoking cessation programs may be health professionals, health educators, or skilled volunteers. Others have a background in substance abuse, are ex-smokers, and those who have witnessed the ill-effects of smoking, such as nurses and respiratory therapists. The American Cancer Society encourages people to make sure that the program leader has had training in smoking cessation counseling.

Some people are interested in alternative therapies, such as acupuncture, laser acupuncture treatment, electrostimulation, and hypnotherapy. Studies have not shown that these alternative or complementary therapies are effective in the treatment of tobacco use. Additionally, an independent review of nine

Table 8   Success Rate of Patients Who Quit Smoking

Type of Clinician	Abstinence Rate (percent)
No clinician	10.2
Self-help	10.9
Non-physician clinician	15.8
Physician clinician	19.9
Two clinician types	23.6
Three or more clinician types	23.0

hypnotherapy trials by the Cochrane Group found insufficient evidence to support hypnosis as a treatment for smoking cessation. Credentialing of these professionals should be carefully investigated. Most accredited acupuncture schools require at least two years of undergraduate study prior to admission; others require students to complete a bachelor's degree. Other training facilities do not require any prior education or experience. It is important to note that there are differences in success rates depending upon the type and number of clinicians utilized (**Table 8**).

56. What is my healthcare professional's role in my smoking cessation?

The role of the healthcare professional is to assist you in selecting the quit assist method that is best for you, teach you tips on how to help yourself with the challenges of quitting, guide you through the steps to stop smoking, and support you during the withdrawal phase. If you are in a smoking cessation group, the counselor or professional will facilitate the group discussion and assist the group members to support each other.

Prior to your decision to quit smoking, your primary healthcare provider should have assessed your smoking history in order to make recommendations about the various resources that are available to help you to quit. Fifty to seventy percent of smokers see their primary healthcare provider each year. All clinicians, particularly primary healthcare providers, are uniquely poised to intervene with patients who use tobacco. Smokers frequently cite a physician's advice to quit as an important motivator for attempting to stop smoking. A physician's advice to quit can increase the odds for success by 30%. A population-based survey found that less than 15% of smokers who saw a physician in the past year were offered assistance to stop smoking and only 3% had a follow-up appointment to address tobacco use. Health professionals should follow the Five A's with every patient:

A physician's advice to quit can increase the odds for success by 30%.

1. Ask about smoking.
2. Advise quitting.
3. Assess willingness to make a quit attempt.
4. Assist in a quit attempt.
5. Arrange a timely follow-up.

57. How much does a smoking cessation program cost?

The cost of smoking cessation programs varies from almost nothing to hundreds of dollars. Many health plans and worksites provide free quit-smoking programs, and some health plans cover the cost of medications to help smokers quit. We recommend that you check with your insurance carrier or employer for information. But before investing your time or money in a program, ask yourself the following questions:

- Is there a cost to me? If so, how much?
- Is the program convenient for me?
- Is the staff well trained and professional?
- Does the program meet my needs?
- What is the success rate of this program?
- What are the program leader's credentials?

58. Does insurance pay for any of the smoking cessation programs or products?

The United States Department of Health and Human Services (DHHS) published recommendations for insurers and managed care organizations to cover tobacco dependence treatments, both counseling and pharmacotherapy, for their subscribers or members of health insurance packages. If you have questions about your insurance coverage, contact your insurance provider and ask them for information. Even if there is no coverage for a smoking cessation program, you should check into payment or partial payment for smoking cessation products.

Medicare covers people who are on Medicare and are diagnosed with a smoking-related illness or are taking medications that may be affected by tobacco. (Question 82 addresses the impact of smoking on the liver.) Medicare will cover up to eight face-to-face visits during a twelve-month period. These visits must be ordered by a physician and provided by a Medicare-recognized practitioner. Medicare will pay 20% of the approved amount after you meet the yearly Part B deductible.

59. What are the benefits of enrolling in a smoking cessation program, and what is the average length of stay of a smoking cessation program?

The success rate increases to 32.5% when a person is enrolled in a more intensive smoking cessation program while also taking anti-smoking addiction medications. The benefits of a smoking cessation program include support, education, and guidance to deal with the psychological and behavioral aspects of nicotine withdrawal. The medications take care of the physiological symptoms of withdrawal.

The American Cancer Society states that there is a strong link between the intensity of an anti-smoking program and success rates. Generally, the more intense the program is, the greater the chance for success. Intensity may include more time in treatment, more or longer sessions, or an increased number of weeks of participation. When considering a program, look for one that has the following:

- The length of each session should be at least 20 to 30 minutes.
- The number of sessions should be at least four to seven.
- The program should last at least two weeks.

Quit-smoking programs that involve more than 90 minutes and up to 300 minutes can increase the success rate of quitting up to 28%, regardless of the method of quitting, and programs that involve eight or more sessions can increase the quit rates up to 24.7%.

Inpatient programs can be found in various parts of the country. Inpatient programs are considered the most intense of all smoking cessation programs. One inpatient smoking cessation program is an eight-day program at the Mayo Clinic in Rochester, Minnesota. This residential program helps severely addicted smokers stop smoking. In a clinical study, it was found that inpatient treatment was more effective for participants who were moderately to severely addicted smokers. Another inpatient program is run by The Seventh Day Adventists, who have a smoking cessation program at the St. Helena Health Center and Hospital, Napa Valley, California. This residential program is over 30 years old. Each stop smoking session lasts a week. During admission, a physical assessment is conducted on each smoker to include lung capacity. Blood and urine tests are done to monitor the adequacy of the dose for those participants using nicotine replacement medications to eliminate withdrawal symptoms. The treatment program is holistic, which includes fluids (namely fruit juices), many fresh fruits and vegetables, and no red meat, chicken, or fish. Massage is combined with exercise in a gym and/or swimming pool, and long walks every morning. An exercise therapist assists participants to increase their endurance, and a nutritionist is available to help participants control the potential weight gain. Group work includes health education and group counseling. There is the option to receive individual counseling, if requested. Both programs are examples of intense smoking cessations programs, which have had a high degree of success.

Joseph's comment:

I find a class like "smoking cessations" a very beneficial way to quit smoking because of the group environment. This allows you to work on the problem with others. Our classes were one hour long, which I felt was a good amount of time to give everyone a chance to share how they were doing and share their tools with other members of the group. Tools included hearing slogans like "You're one away from a pack day" to calling the facilitator if I was having a tough day.

60. How successful are people who quit on their own?

Quitting on one's own may be hard, but it can be done. Many factors contribute to success. First, you must be very motivated to quit. Then you must have made a commitment to quit. To give up cigarettes "cold turkey" means to choose not to use any quit aids that help decrease withdrawal symptoms. Until recently, this was the only option for smokers. The advantage of this method is that the majority of nicotine is out of the body within a few days. Yes, the discomforts can be intense, but the length of time for withdrawal is short. Some smokers think that they do not need to use pharmacotherapy aids and they should just be able to quit by using willpower alone. Other smokers think cold turkey is too extreme. They want the medications to help them through the most difficult time. They choose to avoid the discomfort from the withdrawal symptoms.

Studies have demonstrated that quitting on one's own without the benefits of any therapy results in a success rate of about 4% to 7%. The success rate can be increased to 10% by using over-the-counter (OTC) nicotine replacement therapies. The success rate after a year, using the cold turkey method of quitting is about 4%. At the end of the year, the people who used medications had a success rate equal to the ex-smokers who quit using the cold turkey method.

61. Can smoking cessation be done "one-on-one" with a counselor or health educator, or must it be in a group?

Many find that they are not "group" people and don't enjoy belonging to a group nor participate in any group interactions. For these people, an option is a one-on-one counselor who has a background of either a healthcare provider, healthcare educator, or someone who is skilled in conducting smoking cessation classes. The positive aspect of individual counseling is that individual concerns can be immediately addressed. The negative aspect of one-on-one counseling is that there is no added benefit from the support of a group, whose members are going through a similar ordeal and have many of the same thoughts and feelings. During group counseling sessions, people bounce their thoughts and feelings off each other. For many, the added knowledge of not thinking that he or she is "the only one in the world" going through the withdrawal symptoms is valuable.

Lisa's comment:

The group setting was invaluable for me. I felt that nobody else but my fellow program members really knew what I was going through. Each session, I looked forward to seeing at least one other person still succeeding, as this built up my courage that I, too, could continue to cease smoking.

Joseph's comment:

For me, I learned a tremendous amount from working with the group. I replaced, "I myself will" with "we will" work with others towards a common goal of quitting.

62. What are some of the medication aids, notably the nicotine replacement therapies (NRTs), to smoking cessation?

Nicotine replacement therapies (NRTs) are smoking cessation medicines that release small amounts of nicotine into the bloodstream to help counter cravings and reduce other physical withdrawal symptoms. NRTs are used to slowly wean the smoker off of nicotine. The NRT products contain nicotine, which is equally addictive, but the NRT medications deliver smaller amounts of nicotine than cigarettes and without many of the other harmful effects of tar and carbon monoxide found in cigarettes. Follow the package directions carefully. It is important to first check with your doctor or pharmacist about the interactions of NRT drugs with other drugs you may be taking. Also, check with them about any medical condition that one may have that may restrict the use of an NRT, such as severe cardiovascular disease.

There are currently five forms of nicotine replacement therapies available in the United States: (1) nicotine gum, (2) nicotine patch, (3) nicotine nasal spray, (4) nicotine inhaler, and (5) nicotine lozenge.

1. Nicotine Gum

A physician's prescription used to be required to obtain the gum, but in 1996 the gum became an over-the-counter (OTC) medication. Nicorette is the brand name but there are generic forms of the gum. The manufacturer states that Nicorette allows smokers to self-titrate (up to 24 pieces a day) and it is currently available in six different flavors. The gum allows the nicotine to be absorbed through the mucus membranes of the mouth between the cheek and the gums. It comes in a 4 milligram (mg) dose for those patients who smoke more than 25 cigarettes a day, and a 2 mg dose for those who smoke less than 25 cigarettes a day.

Directions: It is very important you follow the directions on your prescription label carefully and exactly as directed.

One piece of nicotine gum is chewed every one to two hours at first, or it may be chewed when you have the urge to smoke. Chew slowly until you can taste the nicotine or feel a slight tingling in your mouth. Then stop chewing and place (park) the gum between your cheek and gum. When the tingling sensation is almost gone (about 1 minute), start chewing again. Repeat this procedure for about 30 minutes. Do not chew more than one piece of gum at a time, and do not chew one piece after another. Gradually reduce the amount of nicotine gum after two to three months. Reducing the use of nicotine gum over time will help prevent withdrawal symptoms.

Tips to help reduce the use of nicotine gum gradually include:

- Decrease the total number of pieces used per day by about one piece every four to seven days.
- Decrease the chewing time with each piece from the normal 30 minutes to 10 to 15 minutes for 4 to 7 days. Then gradually decrease the total number of pieces per day.
- Substitute pieces of nicotine gum with one or more pieces of sugarless gum for an equal number. Every four to seven days, increase the number of sugarless gum pieces as substitutes for nicotine gum.
- Replace the 4-mg gum with the 2-mg gum and apply the previous steps.
- Consider stopping use of nicotine gum when your craving for nicotine is satisfied by one or two pieces of gum per day.

2. The Nicotine Patch

The patch comes in four main brands: Nicotrol, Nicoderm, Prostep, and Habitrol. All four patches transmit low doses of nicotine to the body throughout the day. Other smoking cessation programs or materials should be used while using the patch.

Directions: It is very important you follow the directions on your prescription label carefully and exactly as directed.

The Nicoderm patch offers a three-step program that can be used for 16 to 24 hours each day. One patch contains 21 mg of nicotine and is recommended for patients who smoke more than 10 cigarettes per day. Another patch contains 14 mg of nicotine and is recommended for patients who smoke less than 10 cigarettes per day. Apply the patch directly to the skin once a day, usually at the same time of day. Apply the patch to a clean, dry, hairless area of skin on the upper chest, upper arm, or hip, as specified by the package directions. Remove the patch from the package, peel off the protected strip, and immediately apply the patch to your skin. The sticky side should touch the skin. Press the patch to the skin by placing the palm of your hand over it for about 10 seconds. Be sure the patch is held firmly in place, especially around the edges. Wash your hands with water only after applying the patch. If the patch falls off or loosens, replace it with a new one. Wear the patch continuously for 16 to 24 hours. The patch may be worn even while showering or bathing. Remove the patch carefully, and dispose of it by folding it in half with the sticky sides touching. After removing the patch, apply the next patch to a different skin area to prevent skin irritation. Nicotine patches may be used from 6 to 20 weeks. A switch to a lower strength patch may be considered after the first two weeks. A gradual reduction to a lower dosage of the patch is recommended so that the amount of nicotine in the system is reduced and consequently, the nicotine withdrawal symptoms will be reduced.

3. Nicotine Nasal Spray

Nicotine nasal spray comes as a liquid to spray into the nose. It should be used along with a smoking cessation program, which may include a support group, counseling, or specific cognitive or behavioral techniques. It allows smokers to cut back on their intake of nicotine gradually. Nicotine is absorbed rapidly through the nasal membranes.

Directions: It is very important you follow the directions on your prescription label carefully and exactly as directed.

To use the nasal spray, follow these steps:

1. Wash your hands.

2. Gently blow your nose to clear your nasal passages.

3. Remove the cap of the nasal spray by pressing in the circles on the side of the bottle.

4. To prime the pump before the first use, hold the bottle in front of a tissue or paper towel.

5. Pump the spray bottle six to eight times until a fine spray appears. Throw away the tissue or towel.

6. Tilt your head back slightly.

7. Insert the tip of the bottle as far as you comfortably can into one nostril, pointing the tip toward the back of your nose. Breathe through your mouth.

8. Pump the spray firmly and quickly one time. Do not sniff, swallow, or inhale while spraying. If your nose runs, gently sniff to keep the nasal spray in your nose. Wait two or three minutes before blowing your nose.

9. Repeat steps six to eight for the second nostril. Replace the cover on the spray bottle.

If you have not stopped smoking at the end of four weeks, talk with your doctor. Your doctor can try to help you understand why you were not able to stop smoking and make plans to try again. Ask your pharmacist or doctor for a copy of the manufacturer's information for the patient. Stay in touch with your doctor. He or she may need to change the doses of your medications once you stop smoking completely. If you continue smoking while using the nicotine nasal spray, you may have some adverse effects. Remember a nicotine overdose can be lethal.

Other Instructions:

-   Handle the bottle with care. If the bottle drops, it may break. If this happens, wear rubber gloves and clean up the spill immediately with a cloth or paper towel. Avoid touching the liquid. Throw away the used cloth or paper towel in the trash. Pick up the broken glass carefully using a broom. Wash the area of the spill a few times.

- If even a small amount of nicotine solution comes in contact with the skin, lips, mouth, eyes, or ears, these areas should be immediately rinsed with water.

4. Nicotine Inhaler

The inhaler should be used with a smoking cessation program, which may include support groups, counseling, or specific cognitive and behavioral therapies. Nicotine oral inhalation comes as a cartridge to inhale by mouth using a special inhaler.

Directions: It is very important you follow the directions on your prescription label carefully and exactly as directed.

Your doctor may increase or decrease your dose depending on your urge to smoke. The inhaler has a plastic mouthpiece with a nicotine plug to deliver the nicotine to the mucous membranes of the mouth. The nicotine in the cartridges is released by frequent puffing over 20 minutes. You may use up a cartridge all at once or puff on it for a few minutes at a time until the nicotine is finished. Try different schedules to see what works best for you.

Read the directions for how to use the inhaler and ask your doctor or pharmacist to show you the proper technique. Practice using the inhaler while in his or her presence. If you continue smoking while using nicotine inhalation, you may experience adverse side effects. Remember: an overdose of nicotine kills. You should know that even though you are using nicotine inhalation, you may have some withdrawal symptoms.

5. Nicotine Lozenge

This is a more recent addition to the growing number of tools to combat nicotine withdrawal symptoms. Slowly allow the lozenge to melt in your mouth.

Directions:

For weeks one to six of treatment, you should use one lozenge every one to two hours. Use at least nine lozenges per day to increase your chances of quitting. During weeks seven to nine, you should use one lozenge every two to four hours. Weeks 10 to 12, you should use one lozenge every four to eight hours. Do not use more than five lozenges in six hours or more than 20 lozenges per day. Do not use more than one lozenge at a time or use one lozenge right after another. Using too many lozenges at a time or one after another can cause side effects such as hiccups, heartburn, and nausea. Do not eat while the lozenge is in your mouth.

Stop using the nicotine lozenges after 12 weeks. After 12 weeks if you still feel the need to use nicotine lozenges, talk to your doctor.

Table 9 summarizes the NRTs presented.

Table 9   Nicotine Replacement Therapies

NRT Medication	FDA Approval and Manufacturer
Nicotine Gum	Approved by the FDA in 1984 in the 2 mg dosage.
	In 1992, the 4 mg dose was approved.
	Manufacturer: GlaxoSmithKline
Nicotine Patch	FDA approval in 1991; approval as an OTC in 1996.
	Manufacturer: GlaxoSmithKline
Nicotine Nasal Spray	FDA approved in 1996.
	Physician's prescription only.
	No generic nasal spray.
	Manufacturer: GlaxoSmithKline
Nicotine Inhaler	Approved by the FDA in 1997.
	No OTC, by prescription only.
	Manufacturer: GlaxoSmithKline
Nicotine Lozenge	Approved by the FDA in 2002.
	Now is an OTC medication. It does not come in a generic form.
	Manufacturer: Commit is lozenges brand name, GlaxoSmithKline

Abbreviations are: FDA, Food and Drug Administration; OTC, over-the-counter (medication).

63. What are the recommendations for when you should take medication in order to quit smoking?

The general recommendation is that all smokers trying to quit should be offered medication. There is compelling evidence that medication aids in abstinence. The evidence is even stronger that medication and counseling are more effective than either alone. For that reason, medication is strongly encouraged. All seven of the FDA-approved medications for treating tobacco use are recommended, including bupropion SR, nicotine gum, nicotine inhaler, nicotine lozenge, nicotine nasal spray, nicotine patch, and varenicline. Additionally, the use of these medications for up to six months does not present a known health risk, and developing dependence on these medications is rare. The higher-dose preparations have been shown to be effective in highly dependent smokers. NRT combinations are especially helpful for highly dependent smokers or those with a history of severe withdrawal. Combining the nicotine patch long-term with nicotine gum, nicotine nasal spray, nicotine inhaler, or bupropion SR, also increases long-term abstinence rates relative to placebo treatments. However, combining varenicline with NRT agents has been associated with higher rates of side effects (such as nausea and headaches). Unfortunately, there are no well-accepted algorithms to guide optimal selection among the first-line medications. Data show that bupropion SR and nicotine replacement therapies, in particular the 4-mg nicotine gum and 4-mg nicotine lozenge, bupropion SR, and nortriptyline appear to be especially effective in treating tobacco-dependent patients diagnosed with depression, but nicotine replacement medications also appear to help individuals with a past history of depression.

That being said, there are some exceptions to that general recommendation. These exceptions are:

There is compelling evidence that medication aids in abstinence.

1. *Women:* Evidence is mixed as to whether NRT is less effective in women than men. The clinician should consider the use of another type of medication with women, such as bupropion or varenicline.

2. *Pregnant women:* These smokers should be encouraged to quit without medication. The studies of medication use are far too small. Bupropion has not been found to be effective at all in pregnant smokers. That being said, one may still recommend medication to this group if, in the clinician's opinion, the benefits outweigh the risks. In pregnant women, for example, the risks of nicotine alone on the mother and the fetus must be weighed against the risks of nicotine, tar and carbon monoxide should the pregnant woman be unable to stop smoking without the benefit of an NRT.

3. *Cardiac patients:* NRT should be used with caution among particular cardiovascular patient groups: those who have had a heart attack within two weeks, those with serious **arrhythmias**, and those with unstable **angina pectoris**.

4. *Light smokers, smokeless tobacco users, and adolescents:* Few studies have been done on these populations to conclude any significant benefit, nor suggest any potential risk. Again, the clinician should weigh the risks against the benefits when considering medications in these populations.

Arrhythmias

Abnormal heart rhythm.

Angina Pectoris

(Also known as angina.) Severe chest pain due to a blockage of blood flow in the arteries of the heart. It is a symptom of an impending heart attack.

64. What are the success rates of the five nicotine replacement therapies alone and in combination with other forms?

The success rates are listed in **Table 10**.

Recent studies have examined the combination of some of the nicotine replacement products and the smoking cessation aids. The FDA has not approved these medications in

Table 10 Success Rates of NRT Medications

NRT Medication	Success Rate
Nicotine Gum	26.1%
Nicotine Patch	23.7%
Nicotine Nasal Spray	26.7%
Nicotine Inhaler	24.8%
Nicotine Lozenge	
2 mg dose	24.2%
4 mg dose	23.6%

combination because of the limited number of efficacy and safety studies. Nevertheless, it is frequently done in practice. Using the patch alone, there is an estimated abstinence rate of 17.4%. By combining the nicotine gum or nicotine lozenge with the patch, the abstinence rate can increase to 28.6%. Therefore, combining the patch with other self-titrating nicotine replacement therapies may be more effective than just using the nicotine patch alone. There is less evidence to support doubling the nicotine patch. In fact, there are warnings against doing so. Combining medications is one of the recommended treatments for those heavy smokers who have difficulty quitting with just the patch and who are being closely monitored by a physician. **Table 11** shows the success rates of NTRs used in combination.

Table 11 Success Rate of NTRs When Used in Combination

Medication	Success Rate
Placebo	13.8%
Patch + ad lib NRT	36.5%
Patch + Bupropion	28.9%
Patch + Inhaler	25.8%
Patch + Nortriptyline	27.3%
Varenicline 2 mg/d	33.2%

Treatment

65. Can I become addicted to any of the drugs used to assist a person to quit smoking?

It is estimated that 1.5 to 2 million Americans try the nicotine gum each year. Thanks to the gum, many people have successfully kicked the cigarette habit. However, some ex-smokers have weaned themselves from one nicotine habit only to pick up a new addiction, but a less risky one. GlaxoSmithKline, manufacturers of Nicorette gum, advises people to stop using the nicotine gum at the end of 12 weeks, and to talk to a doctor if you need to continue to use the gum. But these guidelines haven't stopped some people from using the gum for many months and even years.

In a recent report evaluating data collected by A.C. Nielsen, researchers concluded that 5% to 9% of nicotine gum users relied on nicotine gum longer than the recommended three months. About half of the people in the study used it for six months or longer. In published studies at the Mayo Clinic Nicotine Dependence Center, people have used nicotine gum up to five years without heart or vascular problems. By chewing the gum, the nicotine is delivered slowly through the mucous membranes in the mouth, at much lower levels than the quick-hit surge of nicotine when puffing on cigarettes. At the same time, the gum does not contain any of the cancer-causing substances present in cigarettes. The cancers and vascular diseases associated with smoking develop from the carcinogens, tars, and the carbon monoxide in cigarettes.

66. What is Bupropion SR?

Bupropion is also known as Zyban or Wellbutrin. Zyban is the trade name for the medication when it is prescribed for smoking cessation and Wellbutrin is the trade name for the medication when it is prescribed for depression. It is therefore classified as an antidepressant. Bupropion works by blocking the dopamine transporter pump preventing the transport of dopamine back into the neuron, and thereby increasing the amount of dopamine in the synaptic cleft (see Question 8).

Dopamine is a neurotransmitter found in the brain that is involved in attention, decision making, motor activity, mood, and the generation of psychoses. It is also the major reward chemical thought to be involved in all forms of addiction. (Questions 10 and 32 discuss nicotine's effects on dopamine.) Bupropion comes in two forms of tablets to be taken by mouth: a regular tablet and a sustained-release or extended-release (long-acting) tablet. The regular tablet (Wellbutrin) is usually taken three or four times a day, with doses at least six hours apart. The sustained-release tablet (Wellbutrin SR or Zyban) is usually taken once or twice daily in the morning and afternoon.

Directions:

- Your doctor will probably start you on a low dose of bupropion and gradually increase the dose over time.
- It may take four weeks or longer before you feel the full benefit of bupropion.
- Continue to take bupropion even if you feel well. Do not stop taking bupropion without talking to your doctor.
- Your doctor will probably decrease the dose gradually over a period of two weeks prior to stopping the medication.
- If you forget, skip, or miss a dose, then continue your regular dosing schedule. Do not take a double dose to make up for a missed dose.
- Always allow the full scheduled amount of time to pass between doses of bupropion.

Your doctor may need to change the doses of your medications or monitor you carefully for any pre-existing conditions.

There are a number of conditions for which you should not be taking this medication, including if you have a seizure disorder. If you have anorexia or if you have liver disease you should let your doctor know, as these are general **contraindications** to taking this medication If you experience a serious side effect, you or your doctor should send a report to the Food and Drug Administration's (FDA) Medwatch Adverse Event Reporting

Contraindications

A condition or factor that increases the risk of an adverse event when taking a particular medication or receiving a particular treatment.

program online (at http://www.fda.gov/MedWatch/report. htm) or by phone (1-800-332-1088).

If you are taking the sustained or extended-release tablet, you may notice something that looks like a tablet in your stool. This is just the empty tablet casing and does not mean that you did not get your complete dose of medication.

67. What is Chantix?

Varenicline, known by its trade name Chantix, is the most recent medication that is FDA approved to treat smoking addiction. It is available by prescription only. Currently there is no generic form. Varenicline is a **partial agonist** to a sub-type of the nicotinic acetylcholine receptor. A partial agonist is a compound that both stimulates and inhibits the receptor to a mild degree, thereby eliminating any withdrawal effects associated with smoking cessation, but also eliminating the possibility of deriving any additional pleasure from smoking. It therefore acts like a thermostat, stimulating the receptor when nicotine levels are low and blocking the receptor when nicotine levels are high.

Varenicline was developed by Pfizer through modifying the structure of cytisine, a chemical found in a variety of plants that is known to be a nicotine receptor agonist and has been used as a smoking cessation aid in its own right in Eastern Europe for at least 40 years. Varenicline was fast tracked by the U.S. Food and Drug Administration in February 2006, shortening its approval from 10 to 6 months because of its demonstrated effectiveness in clinical trials and perceived lack of safety issues. The FDA approved varenicline on May 11, 2006, which became available in the U.S. public August 1, 2006, and in the European Union September 29, 2006.

Varenicline comes as a tablet to be taken by mouth. It is usually taken once or twice daily with a full glass of water after eating. Group support programs or individual counseling are strongly recommended as an adjunct to the medication regime.

Partial agonist

A chemical (such as a drug) that can both block and stimulate a receptor depending upon the relative amount of neurotransmitter present in the synaptic cleft. If the amount of neurotransmitter is large, the chemical acts as an antagonist and if the amount of neurotransmitter is low, the chemical acts as an agonist.

Directions:

- Your doctor will probably start you on a low dose of varenicline and gradually increase the dose over the first week of treatment.

- Set a quit date to stop smoking, and start taking varenicline one week before that date. You may continue to smoke during this first week, but stop smoking on the quit date. It may take several weeks for you to feel the full benefit of varenicline.

- You may slip and smoke during your treatment. If this happens, you will still be able to stop smoking.

- Continue to take varenicline for 12 weeks.

- If you have completely stopped smoking at the end of the 12 weeks, your doctor may tell you to take varenicline for another 12 weeks. Continuing to take varenicline may ensure that you will not start to smoke again.

- Once you have stopped smoking, your doctor may need to change the doses of some of your other medications.

- If you have not stopped smoking at the end of 12 weeks, tell your doctor so he or she can help you to understand why you were not able to stop smoking and make plans for you to try to quit again.

Do not use varenicline with other smoking cessation products.

- Varenicline may make you drowsy. Do not drive a car or operate machinery.

- *If you forget a dose:* Take the missed dose as soon as you remember it. However, if it is almost time for the next dose, skip the missed dose and continue your regular dosing schedule. Do not take a double dose to make up for the missed one.

- Do NOT drink alcohol while taking this medication. (However, instructions on the package may not specify if you can drink any alcohol while taking this prescription.)

Call your doctor if you experience any of the following side effects: thinking about harming or killing yourself, planning or trying to do so, or thinking about harming someone else; changes in your usual thoughts, mood, or behavior. **Call your doctor immediately and report it to:** The Food and Drug Administration's (FDA) Medwatch Adverse Event Reporting program online (at http://www.fda.gov/MedWatch/report .htm) or by phone (1-800-332-1088).

68. What is the suicide risk associated with the anti-smoking drug Chantix?

In November 2007, a year and three months after varenicline became available to the American public, the FDA announced it had received reports that patients using it for smoking cessation had experienced several serious psychological symptoms, including suicidal ideation and occasional suicidal and agitated behavior. On February 1, 2008, the FDA issued an alert, noting that "it appears increasingly likely that there is an association between varenicline and serious neuropsychiatric symptoms."

When considering the number of prescriptions, the risks of serious psychological symptoms are extremely low, and the risk that those symptoms will result in death is even lower.

As of February 2008, 491 cases of suicidal thinking or behavior were reported, including 420 in the United States. Thirty-nine of the 491 cases resulted in suicide, including 34 in the United States. More than 6 million people have been prescribed the pill since it was launched. When considering the number of prescriptions, the risks of serious psychological symptoms are extremely low, and the risk that those symptoms will result in death is even lower. When weighing such risks against the risks of continued smoking, varenicline actually ends up being safer than continued tobacco use.

Sorting out the cases individually in order to determine what role, if any, varenicline has in contributing to or even causing these symptoms remains a daunting task. One of the more celebrated cases, the case of Carter Albrecht who was shot by his neighbor after striking his girlfriend and entering his neighbor's house, was probably due to mixing the drug with large amounts of alcohol. Suicidal thinking is a complex behavior with multiple contributing factors, including personality, mood, environment, history, and other substance or prescription medication use. But the end result is often extremely tragic and traumatic, prompting public outcry and a large amount of press. It is important to keep these issues in mind when considering the risks of using this medication against the risks of continuing to smoke.

69. What other non–NRT medication therapies are available, if any?

A number of other medications have been studied, but only two are currently recommended as second-line therapies, should individuals either fail the first-line therapies or experience side effects that contraindicate future use. It is important to remember when selecting medications that prior failure with a medication *does not* predict future failure. Thus, second-line therapies are generally used when first-line therapies are contraindicated or some other compelling clinical reason suggests their trial over a first-line therapy. An example would be for those who have migraines in addition to tobacco dependence, where the clinician would suggest trying nortriptyline as a first-line therapy because it is commonly used to treat migraine headaches. Additionally, there is some evidence demonstrating that women tend to have poor response rates to NRTs and therefore non-NRT medications should be considered, such as bupropion, varenicline, nortriptyline, and clonidine.

The other medications that have been extensively studied, which have *not* been found to be successful include selective serotonin reuptake inhibitors (SSRIs), such as fluoxetine, paroxetine, citalopram, etc., and naltrexone (ReVia). Tobacco dependence is a common problem with depression, and treating the depression can assist the patient in following through with a smoking cessation program. While SSRIs can be used in conjunction with the other smoking cessation medications to treat depression, their use as standalone agents is not effective. Naltrexone has been found to be effective in treating alcoholism in order to assist in abstinence and decrease craving. Naltrexone acts by blocking opiate receptors, but it is not helpful in decreasing craving for cigarettes. Other medications that have not been found to be helpful include benzodiazepines, beta-blockers, silver acetate, and mecamylamine. Mecamylamine is a nicotine antagonist that may prove useful in boosting the effectiveness of antidepressants, but it is too early to tell if this medication will actually pan out.

Two medications that have proven to be effective as second-line therapies include the tricyclic antidepressant, nortriptyline (trade name, Pamelor), and the antihypertensive, clonidine. Nortriptyline blocks the transporter pump and prevents the reuptake of norepinephrine, thus increasing levels of this neurotransmitter in the brain. Norepinephrine release (previously described in Question 9) is stimulated by nicotine, so that nortriptyline may aid as an indirect replacement therapy through this action. Clonidine is a more complicated medication. It generally reduces what is called sympathetic tone—that is, it reduces the "fight or flight response" by reducing the release of norepinephrine. Clonidine is used not only to reduce blood pressure, but also to treat neuropsychiatric conditions such as Tourette's disorder and ADHD (attention deficit hyperactivity disorder, discussed further in Question 83). It is also used to reduce the effects of opiate withdrawal in opiate-dependent patients. Clonidine, in a sense, does the exact opposite of nortriptyline, demonstrating the underlying complexity of nicotine addiction and how oversimplified our current theories are about this drug and its effects on the brain and body.

70. What are the success rates of the non-NRT therapies?

Table 12 shows the success rates of the various non-NRT therapies.

Table 12   Success Rates of Non-Nicotine Replacement Therapies

Non-NRT Medication	Success Rates
Bupropion SR	24.2%
Varenicline 1 mg/d	25.4%
Varenicline 2 mg/d	33.2%
Nortriptyline	22.5%
Clonidine	25.0%
SSRIs	13.7%
Naltrexone	7.3%
Placebo	13.8%

71. What is cognitive behavioral therapy and how is it helpful?

Cognitive behavioral therapy (CBT) involves talking interventions that focus on both thoughts and behaviors. CBT has been shown to be effective with or without the use of medication in smoking cessation. It is a goal-oriented problem-solving approach to overcome distortions resulting from ingrained or automatic thinking that lead to maladaptive behaviors.

Cognitive behavioral therapy is helpful because all smokers develop not only physiological dependency to cigarettes but also psychological and behavioral addictions. The physiological dependency can be dealt with by taking one of the medications for smoking cessation. However, medication cannot take care of the psychological or behavioral addiction. Thoughts and behaviors or addictive habits that people have developed over time are difficult to change. Many people have integrated cigarette smoking into their daily lives (wake up in the morning, smoke; drink coffee, smoke; read the paper, smoke; feed the dog, smoke). Smokers view cigarettes as a friend and a support. There is the "good morning" cigarette, the "pat myself on the back" cigarette, the "stress relief" cigarette, and my "after dinner" cigarette. Consequently, some people need more than just medication. Cognitive behavioral therapy is a great adjunct to pharmacological therapies to ensure a person's success at quitting.

Cognitive behavioral therapy is helpful because all smokers develop not only physiological dependency to cigarettes but also psychological and behavioral addictions.

Treatment

Sykes and Marks from the United Kingdom developed a world-renowned CBT program called *Quit for Life*. It is a two-stage program of reduction and relapse-prevention. The reduction phase aims at a gradual reduction over a 7 to 10 day period. The relapse-prevention phase occurs the week after "D-Day" (that is, the quit day). The goal is to empower a smoker to quit and maintain abstinence.

Smokers may choose the quit methods that are most comfortable for them. A textbook includes a cassette tape, which summarizes the various behavioral and cognitive strategies that participants can select. Handouts for participants include a combination of 30 CBT methods and other materials. A self-help package is provided, which includes:

- A handbook
- Reduction cards
- A progress chart, etc.

Behavioral strategies include:

- Identifying triggers (that is, cues to smoke) and risky situations
- Keeping a smoking diary
- Delaying tactics
- Fading techniques (tapering the nicotine content in NRT medications)
- Behavior substitutes (chewing gum or eating carrot sticks versus smoking cigarettes)
- Positive reinforcements (setting goals and self rewards)
- Self-esteem enhancement
- Coping skills training

The cognitive techniques include:

- Personal responsibility for one's own thoughts
- Learning to change beliefs that prove to be barriers to success

- Disputing irrational thoughts and then replacing them with more positive thoughts
- Homework assignments
- Learning mastery and control
- Cognitive rehearsal (that is, practicing how to deal with risky relapse situations)
- Identifying barriers to successful quitting and how to cope with them

Styles and Marks' studies have shown that *Quit for Life* has quit rates that are five to six times higher than quitting using willpower alone. CBT is another effective method to add to the smoking cessation repertoire of quit programs.

72. Are there 12-step programs for cigarette smokers, like Alcoholics Anonymous (AA)?

Nicotine Anonymous is a form of group therapy. It began in California in 1982, and is similar to Alcoholics Anonymous, the original 12-step, self-help group program. It is based on the assumption that people who share a common problem can collectively support each other to eliminate a destructive behavior and its consequences. The only requirement for belonging to the group is the desire to quit smoking. The emphasis is not only on quitting an addiction but also personal and spiritual growth. The goal is for each member to be completely free of addiction to nicotine. Mutuality, trust, honest sharing, acceptance of self, and other goals are the building blocks for a supportive self-help group. Like other 12-step programs, there is no professional group leader. The 12-step approach develops strong social support networks among participants. Role models who have successfully quit smoking become the leaders and sponsor (mentor) new members. Believing in oneself and in a higher power is strongly encouraged. The concept of a higher power is not faith-based but rather an acceptance of one's own limitations regarding one's ability to change on one's own, thus allowing group members to interpret a stronger outside force that helps to guide them and give them the strength to change according to their own personal beliefs. That outside strength can be the group itself or the extended community. It does not necessarily have to be an abstract being such as God. During the recovery process, group members are encouraged to believe in the power of healing within the group. The 12 steps and 12 traditions for Nicotine Anonymous are similar to Alcoholics Anonymous.

They are as follows:

The Twelve Steps of Nicotine Anonymous

1. We admitted we were powerless over nicotine—that our lives had become unmanageable.

2. We came to believe that a Power greater than ourselves could restore us to sanity.

3. We made a decision to turn our will and our lives over to the care of God as we understand Him.

4. We made a searching and fearless moral inventory of ourselves.

5. We admitted to God, to ourselves, and to another human being the exact nature of our wrongs.

6. We were entirely ready to have God remove all of these defects of character.

7. We humbly asked Him to remove our shortcomings.

8. We made a list of all persons we had harmed, and became willing to make amends to them all.

9. We made direct amends to these people wherever possible, except when to do so would injure them or others.

10. We continued to take a personal inventory and when we were wrong promptly admitted it.

11. We sought through prayer and meditation to improve our conscious contact with God, as we understand Him, praying only for the knowledge of His will for us and the power to carry that out.

12. Having had a spiritual awakening as the result of these steps, we tried to carry this message to nicotine users and to practice these principles in all our affairs.

The Twelve Traditions

1. Our common welfare should come first; personal recovery depends upon Nicotine Anonymous unity.

2. For our group purpose, there is but one ultimate authority—a loving God as He may express Himself in our group conscience. Our leaders are but trusted servants; they do not govern.

3. The only requirement of Nicotine Anonymous membership is the desire to stop using nicotine.

4. Each group should be autonomous except in matters affecting other groups or Nicotine Anonymous as a whole.

5. Each group has but one primary purpose—to carry its message to the nicotine addict who still suffers.

6. A Nicotine Anonymous group ought never endorse, finance, or lend the Nicotine Anonymous name to any related facility or outside enterprise, lest problems of money, property, and prestige divert us from our primary purpose.

7. Every Nicotine Anonymous group ought to be self-supporting, declining outside contributions.

8. Nicotine Anonymous should remain forever non-professional, but our service centers may employ special workers.

9. Nicotine Anonymous, as such, ought never be organized; but we may create service boards or committees, directly responsible to those they serve.

10. Nicotine Anonymous has no opinion on outside issues; hence the Nicotine Anonymous name ought never be drawn into public controversy.

11. Our public relations policy is based on attraction rather than promotion; we need always maintain personal anonymity at the level of the press, radio, TV, and films.

12. Anonymity is the spiritual foundation of all of our traditions, ever reminding us to place principles before personalities.

Self-help groups and psychosocial aftercare groups are highly recommended long-term for people who are at risk for a relapse. Belonging to a group may prevent this common phenomenon.

The success rate of Nicotine Anonymous has not been well documented because Nicotine Anonymous is a self-help group, which is not run by professionals. Some of the data collected to evaluate the effectiveness of a 12-step approach to smoking cessation was conducted at an inpatient program run by the Palo Alto Veterans Administration Hospital in California. The smoking cessation program, which was run by professionals, used a 12-step approach. A study compared the hospital-based 12-step program with another inpatient program, which used cognitive behavioral therapy as the approach to smoking cessation. The results showed that over 45% of the men enrolled in the 12-step program were abstinent one year after discharge, compared to 36% of the men who received cognitive behavioral therapy.

73. Why is group therapy as important as anti-tobacco drug therapy?

Group therapy is a frequent intervention used in smoking cessation programs.

Group intervention is not necessarily the most effective method of quitting when it is the only method used; however, it is effective in combination with other smoking cessation tools, including medications. Group programs teach people to recognize problems that occur while quitting. Group members

Table 13 Successful Abstinence Rates by Type of Therapy

Format	Estimated Abstinence Rate
No format	10.8%
Self-help	12.3%
Telephone counseling	13.1%
Group counseling	13.9%
Individual counseling	16.8%
Two formats	18.5%
Three or more formats	23.2%
0–1 Counseling sessions	21.8%
2–3 Counseling sessions	28.0%
4–8 Counseling sessions	26.9%
More than 8 counseling sessions	32.5%
Counseling without medication*	14.6%
Counseling with medication*	22.1%

* Data cannot be compared as they are from a different set of research.

offer emotional support and encourage each other to reach for success, which many people find helpful. Studies have demonstrated differences in abstinence success rates depending upon the type of therapy utilized as well as whether or not it is used in combination with medication therapy. **Table 13** illustrates those differences. (It is important to note that the medication and counseling statistic is from a different set of studies, and therefore one cannot compare that number against any of the other numbers as denoted by the asterisk [*].)

74. Are there herbal remedies for smoking cessation?

Thousands of people are looking for alternative approaches to smoking cessation. As a result, non-traditional quit smoking methods look attractive to many who do not want to take medications or to participate in traditional programs used to stop smoking. These alternatives are known as Complementary and Alternative Medicine (CAM). The U.S. Department of Health and Human Services (DHHS) conducted a meta-analysis that determined alternative therapies such as hypnosis, acupuncture, electrostimulation, and laser treatments were not effective in tobacco cessation. If you decide on herbal medicines, discuss your plan with your doctor, pharmacist, or a holistic health practitioner.

Herbal Remedies

All of the following herbs that will be discussed have been used as aids for smoking cessation. Herbs have been used traditionally in Eastern medicine for years but have been introduced to Americans only recently. There are herbal teas as well as pills that are available over-the-counter (OTC) at health food stores.

Ginseng

Ginseng is a root that has been made into a medication, which has been used historically in Chinese medicine for 7000 years. It is grown in the Far East as well as the United States. Ginseng can be eaten raw or prepared using various methods. The best way to prepare it is to brew it into a tea. Ginseng is purported to reduce stress, improve cognitive performance, boost energy, enhance memory, and stimulate the immune system. Many of these effects are similar to the effects of nicotine. Studies conducted in China reported that ginseng increased the activity of the brain's neurotransmitters.

Kava

Kava is a sacred drink to many Pacific Islanders. Kava is purported to relieve anxiety that is associated with the withdrawal symptoms of a variety of addictive drugs including nicotine and alcohol. Kava is non-addictive and is also an appetite suppressant. One of the chemicals found in kava inhibits the enzyme monoamine oxidase-B (MAO-B), which is also inhibited by the antidepressants Nardil and Parnate. Inhibiting MAO increases the neurotransmitters dopamine and norepinephrine in the brain, which may explain why kava is thought to have smoking cessation properties. However, neither Nardil nor Parnate are believed to be safe or effective in treating tobacco dependence, and they are far more potent MAO inhibitors than kava. Kava is contraindicated in all patients taking antidepressant medications.

The therapeutic uses of kava are as follows:

- Relieves anxiety and stress and the ensuing depression
- Is a muscle relaxant
- Is a diuretic and anti-inflammatory medication
- Is an anti-convulsant
- Protects against strokes
- Is a mild analgesic
- Is a mild anesthetic
- Is a topical antifungal medication

Lobelia

Lobelia also has been called the *Indian Tobacco* or the *puke-weed*. It is a purgative used in small doses as an expectorant to treat respiratory problems; in large doses it is used as an emetic (it makes you vomit) to treat food poisoning. It grows all over North America. It has nicotine-like properties in that it is both a stimulant and a relaxant. In small doses, lobelia can have a soothing, sedative effect. It can calm the jittery nerves of someone who is withdrawing from nicotine. Thus, if lobelia is taken during smoking withdrawal, the cravings will be reduced. If one smokes a cigarette while taking lobelia, however, the smoker may become nauseated and may vomit. It also may have mild antidepressant effects, which helps with the initial sadness during nicotine withdrawal.

Precautions: It is contraindicated to take lobelia during pregnancy, if you have low blood pressure, if you get easily nauseated, if you are taking blood pressure medications, if you are a diabetic, or if you are already on potassium replacement therapy, diuretics, or corticosteroids. If you are taking aspirin and nonsteroidal anti-inflammatory drugs (NSAIDs), the combination can increase the risk of a toxic reaction.

75. How many times does a typical smoker quit throughout his or her life?

Many attempts at quitting are often the norm. Occasionally you will find someone who threw the cigarettes out and never went back. That is atypical for most smokers. Research shows that 70% of smokers want to quit, 81% of smokers have tried to quit at least once, 35% try to quit each year, and quitting may require more than 10 attempts before becoming successful. Only about 7% of smokers attempting to quit remain smoke-free at the end of one year. This is exactly why tobacco dependence should be thought of as a chronic relapsing condition, and adding the various medications and support groups available can increase the success rates for quitting.

Only about 7% of smokers attempting to quit remain smoke-free at the end of one year.

76. What can I do to avoid "triggers"?

Triggers are the environmental stimuli that are associated with smoking and serve to support the ongoing habit. A trigger prompts you to reach for a cigarette. Some of the most common triggers for smoking are things such as stress, coffee, and alcohol. Other triggers include:

- The morning routine
- Certain people, often smoking buddies or a spouse
- Driving
- Finishing a meal
- Watching TV
- Talking on the phone
- Post coitus
- Boredom
- Finishing something
- Breaks at work or after work
- Feeling anxious, tense, angry, or lonely

Whatever the triggers may be, it's important to make note of them. If you prepare for your triggers, you can handle them better. Avoiding triggers, at least until you are more secure as a nonsmoker, will help in the process. Triggers can overwhelm the unprepared quitter.

Try the "4 Ds":

- Drink plenty of water, between six and eight glasses per day.

- Delay the impulse to smoke for three to seven minutes. The urge should pass.

- Do something else that will take your mind elsewhere.

- Deep breathe.

It is important to drink lots of fluids, eat right, and get enough sleep. A poor diet and the lack of a good night's sleep can decrease your resistance to triggers. Cognitive behavioral therapy and support groups also help to both identify the triggers and assist in developing coping strategies when one is confronted with a trigger (see Questions 71–73).

Lisa's comment:

During the first days after quitting, I experienced a mysterious and disturbing phenomenon whereby I received repetitive images of my right arm (I am right-handed) that kept swinging up to my face holding a lit cigarette. I did not want a cigarette; however, I told my therapist that I could not imagine going through the rest of my life with this image "assaulting" me. She told me to vocalize my determination to quit and that my subconscious would listen. Every time the image jumped up, I loudly spoke out "I do not want a cigarette. I have a higher goal in mind, and that is to live my life as a nonsmoker; smoking a cigarette is an obstacle to reaching my goal." It's truly amazing how quickly this worked and how the appearance of the image began to decrease in frequency, until it disappeared altogether. The images stopped in a few days after this method.

77. What is the difference between a "slip" and a "relapse"?

Two terms are used when talking about getting a person back on track to quitting: slips and relapses. A slip is when you have a cigarette or two after you have quit smoking. It is not uncommon for people who are trying to quit to have an occasional slip. Because smoking can be so automatic, you may not even be consciously aware that you've smoked until after you've finished. A slip or two does not mean that you have failed. If you slip, the best thing to do is get back on track immediately. Look at the trigger that led to the slip and figure out how to handle it differently next time. A slip will not prevent you from quitting successfully. It is all part of learning to quit smoking.

Tips for preventing slips:

- Reinforce why you want to quit.
- Think of all the hard work you've done so far. Would you ever want to repeat it again?
- Continue positive self-talk; do not get discouraged.
- Say mantras such as, "One away from a pack a day."
- Get help and support from friends.
- Ride out the temptation. The urge usually lasts only three to seven minutes. Deep breathe during the tempting moments.
- Look at what caused you to smoke and how you plan on getting back on track.
- Develop a plan to deal with the situation in the future.

A relapse is when you start smoking again daily. A relapse will not prevent you from quitting sometime in the future. Quitting smoking is a process, and most people make more than one quit attempt before they stop for good. Don't feel discouraged. As long as you learn something positive with each quit attempt, you will be further ahead than before your first attempt. You can overcome relapses by:

Treatment

- Not beating yourself up or losing hope.

- Thinking of the relapse as a learning experience and one more step in your journey to becoming smoke-free.

- Planning a new quit attempt right away, including developing a plan to prevent relapse.

- Being aware of the people, places, situations, thoughts, and emotions that trigger your urge to smoke.

- Planning ahead what you will do to cope with each trigger. You should continue to be aware of your triggers for a long time after you quit. Some situations, especially unexpected ones such as crises, can catch you by surprise. If you figure out ahead of time how you will deal with difficult situations, you are more likely to stay quit.

78. Is it ever too late to quit?

Many people will ask, "why should I bother quitting, the damage is probably already done?" No matter how old you are or how long you've smoked, quitting will help to prolong your life. (Questions 37 and 38 detail the benefits of quitting.) People who stop smoking at age 50 statistically can cut their risk of dying in the next 15 years compared to those who continue to smoke.

No matter how old you are or how long you've smoked, quitting will help to prolong your life.

A prospective study of the early stages of chronic obstructive pulmonary disease (COPD) found that forced expiratory volume in one second (**FEV1**) falls gradually over a lifetime, but in most nonsmokers, clinically significant airflow obstruction never develops. In susceptible people, however, smoking may cause irreversible changes in lung function. If a susceptible smoker stops smoking, then he or she will probably not recover all of their lung function, but over time the average rate of loss of FEV1 may revert to near normal. By screening smokers' lung function when they are middle aged, COPD can be prevented. Those with reduced function should be persuaded to stop smoking immediately.

FEV1 (Forced Expiratory Volume in One Second)

Part of a set of measures collectively called pulmonary function tests that allow physicians to measure lung function. FEV 1 measures the total volume of air exhaled in one second.

Below is a list of the health benefits of quitting smoking and the timeline for recovering your health:

- **20 minutes after quitting:** Your heart rate and blood pressure drop.

- **2 weeks to 3 months after quitting:** Your circulation improves and your lung function increases.

- **1 year after quitting:** The risk of coronary heart disease is half that of a smoker's.

- **5 to 15 years after quitting:** The risk of a stroke is reduced to that of a nonsmoker.

- **5 to 10 years after quitting:** The lung cancer death rate is about half that of a continuing smoker's. The risk of cancer of the mouth, throat, esophagus, bladder, cervix, and pancreas decreases.

- **15 years after quitting:** The risk of coronary heart disease is that of a nonsmoker's.

The rewards for not smoking continue throughout the years, prolonging your life and enhancing your day to day living, doing what is socially acceptable and ensuring the health of others by not exposing them to secondhand smoke.

79. What are the success rates of smokers who quit "cold turkey" and those who quit by participating in a smoking cessation program?

Success rates of smoking cessation methods vary from method to method, depending upon the reporter and his or her mission. Estimates of success rates for the "cold turkey" method (stopping without any medication or other therapy) are between 4% and 7%. Cold turkey results in the lowest rates of successful quitting, but it does achieve the lowest nicotine blood levels within the shortest period of time, compared to nicotine replacement therapies (NRTs). The best data come from the studies on the FDA-approved medications; the most inadequate data about success rates are the results of studies that involve the herbal medicines. The success rates of the NRTs range from 17% to 49%. The success rates of the antidepressants, bupropion and Chantix range between 30.5% for bupropion and 70.5% for Chantix. Successful outcomes of group interventions are extremely rare if used as the only intervention, but in combination with NRT and other therapeutic measures, success rates are greatly improved. Group counseling is frequently recommended for long-term maintenance and relapse prevention because the success rates of continuing to remain smoke-free are better if there is continuing support. Hypnosis and other alternative interventions are not well documented by long-term systematic control studies and therefore cannot be recommended.

Treatment

PART FIVE

Associated Conditions

What are the medical consequences of tobacco use?

How does smoking affect the liver?

Are there any health benefits to tobacco or nicotine?

More . . .

80. What are the medical consequences of tobacco use?

Tobacco use kills an estimated 440,000 U.S. citizens each year, which is more than alcohol, cocaine, heroin, homicide, suicide, car accidents, fires, and AIDS combined. Since 1964, more than 12 million Americans have died prematurely from tobacco, and another million U.S. tobacco users alive today will most likely die of a tobacco-related illness. Tobacco use harms every organ in the body. It accounts for about one-third of all cancer-related deaths and for a host of other diseases such as leukemia, cataracts, lung diseases of all types, vascular disease, and the body's ability to successfully heal and fight infections of all types.

Tobacco use harms every organ in the body.

The overall rates of death from cancer are twice as high among smokers as nonsmokers. Foremost among the cancers caused by tobacco use is lung cancer. Cigarette smoking has been linked to about 90% of all lung cancer cases and is the number one cancer killer of both men and women. Today, the rate of lung cancer in women exceeds breast cancer. Smoking is also associated with cancers of the lips, mouth, pharynx, larynx, esophagus, stomach, colon, pancreas, cervix, kidney, and bladder.

Gender Differences in Diseases Found in Smokers

Males

Men have been smoking since the Virginia colony started growing tobacco for American and European consumption. The overall rate of men who smoke is higher than women, as are the death rates. However, currently the rates of male smokers and deaths due to smoking have declined since the *Surgeon General's Report* was published in 1964 (see Question 21). Older men are more likely to be former smokers than older women, who have difficulty quitting.

Females

Because women find it harder to quit than men, the incidence of lung cancer in women has been increasing both in North America and Europe. A Swiss research team concluded that the rate of smoking and deaths due to smoking among women has yet to reach its peak. In time, female smokers will out-number male smokers.

Differences in Gender-Specific Health Risks

The risks for males who smoke are decreased fertility and erectile dysfunction. Women over 35 who are smokers and are on birth control pills are at a greater risk for developing blood clots, which may cause a heart attack or a stroke. It is strongly advised that women who are on birth control pills should stop smoking. Other risks include potential physical problems, which are related to reproduction, pregnancy, and mothering. Smoking causes premature aging. Many women who smoke are prone to ectopic pregnancies. Smoking may cause early menopause.

Men and Women

Smoking is the leading cause of death among both American and European men and women. Diseases related to smoking are preventable. Smoking causes about 90% of the early deaths in men and about 80% of female deaths.

81. Can you list all of the specific diseases associated with smoking?

Cardiovascular:

- Ischemic heart disease
- Stroke
- Peripheral vascular disease
- Abdominal aortic aneurysm
- Microvascular disease affecting end organs (examples include exacerbation of Raynaud syndrome, poor wound healing after major surgery, erectile dysfunction)

Respiratory:

- Chronic obstructive pulmonary disease (COPD)
- Community acquired pneumonia
- Poor asthma control
- Emphysema

Cancer:

- Lung cancer
- Cancer of the mouth, throat, and esophagus; pancreatic cancer, colon cancer
- Cervical cancer, vulvar cancer, and contributes to abnormal Pap smears
- Renal cell carcinoma, bladder cancer
- Leukemia

Reproductive:

- Erectile dysfunction (via micro vascular disease)
- Lowered sperm counts
- Miscarriages
- Ectopic pregnancies

Other:

- Macular degeneration
- Periodontal disease
- Osteoporosis
- Peptic ulcers
- Burns
- Hepatic: Stimulation of liver metabolism of other drugs resulting in a loss of their effectiveness; acceleration of fibrosis in hepatitis

All of these diseases and conditions are a result of tobacco use and not nicotine. Nicotine is merely the major chemical involved in forming the addiction to tobacco. It is the cause of the disease of dependency. While it also exacerbates the cardiovascular effects of underlying vascular disease, because of its stimulatory effects on heart rate and blood pressure by constricting the blood vessels and stimulating the sympathetic nervous system, it does not directly cause vascular disease. It is all of the other ingredients, which are not in themselves addictive that lead to the long list of other diseases mentioned above. These other ingredients are discussed in greater detail in Questions 12 and 13.

82. How does smoking affect the liver?

The liver's primary responsibility is removing toxins from the body. It does this by filtering the blood to separate substances that are good for the body from those that are toxic to the body. The more toxins that are filtered, the less efficient the liver is at performing this duty. Cigarette smoking induces certain **cytochrome P450 enzymes** in the liver, causing them to accelerate their activity, thus breaking down chemicals at a faster rate. As a result, medications that are eliminated by those enzymes are also eliminated at a faster rate, decreasing their levels in the body and rendering them less effective. This may affect the dose of medication required to treat a particular disease. It is important to let your doctor know that you are smoking, as this may prompt her or him to alter the dose of a medication if it is not working.

Despite this observation, as yet there is no conclusive evidence that tobacco use has an adverse effect on the liver, although cigarettes may worsen the course of alcoholic liver disease. Additionally, other studies have suggested that tobacco smoking may promote the progression of fibrosis in hepatitis C patients, accelerating the disease process, although this has been less extensively studied than alcohol. The accelerated fibrosis associated with cigarette smoking may be triggered by lower oxygen levels on a microvascular level in smokers. Therefore, it is recommended that people with liver disease refrain from using these forms of tobacco as well.

Cytochrome P450 enzymes

A group of enzymes found in the liver that function to break down chemicals for elimination from the body. These chemicals include but are not limited to medications. Some medications can block these enzymes while other medications or drugs, such as nicotine, can induce or accelerate these enzymes.

83. Are there any health benefits to tobacco or nicotine?

Tobacco, when used for specific purposes has long been considered to be safe, if not healthy in its history. Native Americans understood and appreciated its toxicity when used excessively either in quantity or frequency. Limited to specific ceremonies and to the pharmacopeia of the Medicine Men and Women, tobacco was regarded as a perfectly acceptable healing herb. It was used as a pain killer for earache and toothache and occasionally as a poultice. It was used by the desert Indians to be a cure for colds, especially if mixed with the leaves of the small desert sage, or the root of Indian balsam or cough root, which was thought to be particularly good for asthma and tuberculosis. In addition it was often eaten to be used as a purgative or in enemas. In 1571, a Spanish doctor wrote a book about the history of medicinal plants of the New World, including tobacco, which was thought to cure 36 health problems. When tobacco first arrived in the Ottoman Empire, it attracted the attention of doctors and became a commonly prescribed medicine for many ailments. Until the first *Surgeon General's Report* in 1964, tobacco companies often enlisted the support of physicians to promote smoking. One can see 1950s TV commercials and magazine ads with physicians, glamorous movie and TV stars, and even athletes promoting its use.

While the idea of tobacco conferring any health benefits today seems almost ludicrous, the issue of nicotine's positive impact on health remains hotly investigated. A number of people with neuropsychiatric conditions tend to smoke heavily. These conditions include attention deficit hyperactivity disorder (ADHD), depression, and schizophrenia. All of these conditions share the symptom of inattention as an underlying problem. Nicotine, as a stimulant, impacts dopamine, a major neurotransmitter in the maintenance of attention. Studies using functional magnetic resonance imaging (fMRI) in smokers demonstrate that nicotine clearly improved the activity of areas of the brain known to be involved in attention. In addition, researchers have found genes regulating specific nicotine receptors in schizophrenics to be reduced. A recent study conducted by Robert Freedman, MD, at the University of Colorado and published in the June 2006 issue of *Archives of Psychiatry*, tested a drug that targets that specific nicotine receptor. In that small study, the drug, known as **DMXB-A**, was found to improve certain cognitive symptoms in schizophrenia. Paul Newhouse at the University of Vermont is investigating nicotine and nicotine-related drugs in ADHD.

DMXB-A

A drug that activates the alpha-7 subtype of the nicotine receptor and is being used experimentally to improve cognition in patients with Alzheimer's disease and schizophrenia.

Smokers appear to have lower rates of neurodegenerative disorders, such as Alzheimer's disease, Parkinson disease, multiple sclerosis, and Huntington chorea. This may be due to the fact that nicotine boosts the neurotransmitters dopamine and acetylcholine, which play roles in these conditions. Newhouse is also experimenting with using nicotine patches to treat mild cognitive impairment, a possible precursor to Alzheimer's disease.

Nicotine also plays a role in obesity and pain. Nicotine historically was used to treat toothache. In animals it has been demonstrated to provide modest pain relief. Recently, epibatidine, a drug extracted from a South American frog that acts on nicotine receptors, has been found to be 200 times more potent than morphine in blocking pain in animals. Other researchers have demonstrated that intranasal nicotine use reduces the need for morphine in some postoperative patients. Nicotine is also being investigated in weight control, a problem every ex-smoker struggles with soon after they quit. Nicotine appears to up-regulate certain hormones that play a role in appetite regulation so that appetite is suppressed by their increase. In one study on rats, the animals were able to lose not only their weight, but also 20% of their body fat. Nicotine appears to affect all molecules that are known to influence weight, which may be one of the earliest nicotine-based treatments that are nonsmoking related.

Before you jump to a nicotine replacement therapy to treat or "prevent" any of these conditions, it is important to remember that the research is ongoing and none of the benefits listed here are either well validated or risk-free. The risks of nicotine are well known, particularly when used in excess, and most notably include cardiorespiratory collapse and death, aside from the risks associated with any stimulant that is addictive.

PART SIX

Special Populations

What are the differences in the rates of tobacco use among different ethnic groups?

How can smoking affect my baby during pregnancy?

What are the rates of smoking between socioeconomic groups and educational levels?

More . . .

84. What are the differences between men and women regarding rates of tobacco use, history of tobacco use, and their health risks?

There are many differences between men and women regarding smoking and tobacco addiction. Men start smoking earlier than women, usually in their early teens, inhale more deeply, but have an easier time quitting. They often quit while they are still relatively young. Women, on the other hand, start smoking later, usually in their late teens or early twenties, smoke less, do not inhale as deeply as men, tend to smoke "lighter" or filtered cigarettes, but have a much harder time quitting.

Both physiological and social factors may contribute to a woman's greater dependence on nicotine. Physiological factors include the body weight/mass index (women carry more body fat than men). When examining social factors related to gender differences of smoking behaviors, male smokers tend to be loners while female smokers tend to gather in groups and socialize while they smoke. When it comes to treatment, women using nicotine gum therapy reported greater withdrawal symptoms than men. (See Question 63 for more information about medication therapy for women.) More research is needed to better understand such gender differences. Results from gender-based studies might provide guidelines that tailor effective smoking cessation treatment strategies for each gender.

Men start smoking earlier than women, usually in their early teens, inhale more deeply, but have an easier time quitting.

85. What are the differences in the rates of tobacco use among different ethnic groups?

Native Americans and Alaskan Natives

Today there are 562 federally recognized Native American tribes in the United States. Each tribe has its own language, customs, and rituals, particularly regarding the use of tobacco. Prevalence rates of smoking vary among tribes from region to region. The highest tobacco use is in Alaskan Natives; and the next region with a high rate of smoking is the Northern Plains tribes, while the lowest rate of tobacco use is found in the Southwestern tribes.

Native Americans have a high rate of addiction to alcohol and drugs of all types, including tobacco. Alcoholism among Native Americans may be due to a genetic vulnerability. Drinking alcohol and smoking are behaviors that frequently go hand-in-hand. Thus, alcoholism may be a contributory factor in the rate of heavy smoking among Native Americans and Alaskans. Poverty and a lack of education are also strongly associated with smoking. Native Americans tend to be less educated and tend to be poorer than other U.S. ethnic minorities. Many live at or below the poverty line because of a lack of economic opportunities on reservations. A higher percentage of smokers exist across all socioeconomic groups. Forty-one to forty-two percent of Native Americans and Alaskan natives smoke, which is a much higher statistic than all other Americans. Consequently, there is a high mortality rate from smoking among them, two times greater than among other Americans. Native Americans frequently die of cardiovascular diseases, lung cancer, and cancers of the **bronchus** and trachea.

Cultural and Spiritual Factors

Tobacco was used for spiritual, social, and political purposes. Tobacco also was used for medicinal healing and in agriculture. Tobacco is considered a sacred gift and has played an important role in Native American culture throughout history. (Questions 2 and 3 discuss the many uses of tobacco.) During the fur trading era of the seventeenth and eighteenth centuries, traditional uses of tobacco became combined with commercial uses. The importance of tobacco as central to many sacred ceremonial events has diminished since Indians became acculturated into the dominant European culture. The current use of tobacco does not resemble how it was used in the past.

Bronchus

The large airway of the lungs. No gas exchange between the lungs and the bloodstream occurs here.

Native American Women

The rate of smoking is also higher among Native American women (34.5%) than the rest of American women. This percentage is even higher among those living in the Northern Plains states (43.5%). Pregnant women who are smokers tend to continue to smoke while pregnant, which results in underweight newborns or miscarriages.

Native American Teens

The number of Native American teens who smoke is more than double the number of all other high school students from other ethnic groups. Indian Reservations are considered sovereign states and therefore are not subject to state laws that prohibit the sale of tobacco products to minors. Indian nation states do not levy taxes on cigarette sales, which may contribute to the higher prevalence of smoking. Easy access to low-cost tobacco products probably contributes to the numbers of teens who use tobacco products.

Besides smoking, the use of smokeless tobacco is more prevalent among Native American teens. A significant number of young Native Americans age 15 to 24 use smokeless tobacco products. Fourteen percent of males and 2% of females use smokeless tobacco, compared to 5.2% of American males and 1.5% of American females from other ethnic groups.

The Elderly

The rate of Native American smokers who are over 65 is the highest in the nation, 20% higher than in the general population. As a result, tobacco use has resulted in a high rate of tobacco-related diseases among Native Americans, which kills close to 10,000 Native Americans yearly. This is double the death rate for all other Americans dying from tobacco use.

Prevention and Smoking Cessation Programs

Concerted efforts by the Indian Health Service and the American Cancer and Lung Associations are underway to assist Native American communities to establish smoking cessation and primary prevention programs. Prevention strategies involve peer-to-peer counseling and changes in advertising and access to tobacco products. Teens are trained by tribal leaders to be peer counselors. Native American communities have passed anti-tobacco policies to reduce the incidence of smoking and the exposure of their citizens to secondhand smoke. Billboards advertising tobacco products are banned. Culturally sensitive smoking prevention materials are handed out during community events, such as pow-wows, potlatches, health fairs, rodeos, sporting events, and festivals. School programs similar to other school programs on tobacco prevention are taught in the public and private schools. Media campaigns targeting high-risk youth are aired on the radio and TV to reduce the initiation of new smokers.

Hispanics

Among Hispanic smokers living on the U.S. mainland, Cubans comprise 61.5% of the smokers and Puerto Rican Americans amount to 4.2% of the smokers. Mexican Americans are lighter smokers than other Hispanics, Anglos, and Blacks. More Hispanic men smoke than women, by 21.1%. Those Hispanics who do smoke are able to quit more easily than their non-Hispanic counterparts. Many of the women stop smoking during pregnancy. If Hispanic women smoke at all, they begin later in life. Generally, all Hispanics consume fewer cigarettes each day compared to other ethnic groups. Twenty-two percent of Hispanic high school students are smokers. Many of the Hispanic male smokers are among the more poorly educated, and have jobs such as day laborers or migrant workers. Being Hispanic appears to be a protection against a smoking addiction.

Asian Americans

Asian Americans are among the smallest group of smokers in the United States. However, even though the overall rates of smoking among Asian Americans are low, the rate of smoking among Asian American men is significantly higher than the rate of smoking among Asian American women. Only 13.3% of Asian Americans currently smoke, and of those who do smoke, only 6.1% of the smokers are women.

African Americans

During the twentieth century, African Americans began smoking later than Caucasians in the history of tobacco use. Many black women have never smoked, but men who are poor, uneducated, and work in low paying jobs have a higher rate of smoking than their better educated and employed counterparts. By the 1960s, rates of smoking among blacks and whites were similar. Mentholated cigarettes were heavily advertised in the black media as being safer (Kools, Newport, Salems). As rates of smoking began to decline in the 1970s and early 1980s, advertising agencies for the tobacco companies began to devote more money to promote sales among black teens. Billboards targeting African American communities were concentrated in poorer urban neighborhoods. A 1987 survey of St. Louis found that black neighborhoods had three times as many billboards as white neighborhoods advertising cigarettes.

Disproportionately, black men are more likely to develop lung cancer than white men, even though black men smoke fewer cigarettes. African Americans may have metabolic differences that are genetically based, which leads to an inability to detoxify the carcinogens in tobacco. The menthol in mentholated cigarettes has numbing properties so that the smoker inhales the smoke more deeply into the lungs. African Americans' preference for mentholated cigarettes may explain why they are more prone to lung cancer.

86. *How can smoking affect my baby during pregnancy?*

Smoking during pregnancy puts both the mother and baby at risk. Smokers have a miscarriage rate that is twice as high as that of nonsmokers. These miscarriages are often genetically normal fetuses. Pregnant women who smoke are twice as likely to experience placental complications such as placenta previa, a condition where the placenta grows too close to the opening of the uterus, sometimes necessitating a caesarean section; placental tears, where the placenta prematurely separates from the wall of the uterus; and premature rupture of the membranes before labor begins. All of these can contribute to miscarriages.

When a pregnant mother smokes, the child is affected by the toxic compounds of nicotine and by the lack of oxygen to all the cells in the body, which may not only affect the child's development in the womb, but also may affect the child's later growth and development. There is some evidence that smoking interferes with a mother's hormonal balance during pregnancy, which then affects the baby. A pregnant woman who smokes is at greater risk of having a premature baby, a prenatal death, or an underweight baby. There is also speculation that smoking may contribute to sudden infant death syndrome (SIDS) during infancy. Some researchers think the risk that an infant will die of SIDS is double the risk when the mother is a smoker. There is not only a higher incidence of SIDS among babies whose mother smoked during pregnancy but also babies whose mothers smoked around them immediately after birth. The following is a list of the effects of nicotine on the fetus, the neonate, and the overall development of the child.

When a pregnant mother smokes, the child is affected by the toxic compounds of nicotine and by the lack of oxygen to all the cells in the body, which may not only affect the child's development in the womb, but also may affect the child's later growth and development.

The Fetus (the Unborn Baby)

- Intrauterine growth retardation (slow growth)
- The baby may be small and underweight
- Microcephaly (small head and brain)

- Premature birth
- High fetal mortality

Neonate (the Newborn)

- May be "jittery"
- Have poor sucking or feeding responses
- SIDS
- Birth defects

Early Childhood

- The child may be slow to learn and have school problems.
- Many of these children are diagnosed with ADHD.
- If microcephaly occurs, then the child will be mentally retarded.
- Conduct disorder (anti-personality disorder) and other behavior problems are more likely.
- Many have respiratory problems and/or allergies, such as asthma.

If the mother continues to smoke after the baby is born or relapses after having stopped smoking during pregnancy, the infant will continually be exposed to secondhand smoke, which may cause respiratory problems, allergies, and ultimately all the other conditions associated with secondhand smoking (see Questions 21 and 80). Many mothers relapse somewhere within the first six months after the birth of the baby.

The following factors contribute to a mother relapsing after stopping during pregnancy:

- Exposure to other mothers who are smoking
- Deciding not to breast-feed
- Heavy smoking prior to the pregnancy
- The stress and adjustment to motherhood and a new identity

87. How does smoking affect breast milk?

It is better not to smoke if breast-feeding for several reasons. First and foremost, an infant is exposed to both nicotine as well as other tobacco toxins through the breast milk. Some babies may develop signs of nicotine intoxication if the mother smokes heavily, including nausea, vomiting, and diarrhea. Second, the tobacco toxins passed through breast milk are greater than exposure through secondhand smoke, which means one is more than doubling a baby's exposure to tar and nicotine by exposing the baby through two routes. Third, tobacco negatively effects colostrum, the most nutritious component of early breast milk, rich in **immunoglobulin**, and part of a mother's body's immune system, which helps the infant fight infection. Fourth, smoking hinders the mother's let down of milk. Finally, smoking curtails breast milk production. The baby may then not get enough milk and may show signs of hunger and dehydration.

88. What are the differences in the smoking habits at different ages, from children to the elderly?

Children

One-quarter of teen smokers started smoking when they were under 10 years old. One in eight middle school children have tried smoking. A recent study examined the relationship between ADHD and smoking. Young adult smokers who had been diagnosed as having ADHD as young children reported that they started smoking before the age of 10 (see Question 83 for further information on ADHD). This group of young adults reported when they were children, they smoked several packs per day. Socially isolated children often smoke in order to become part of a group.

Immunoglobulin

An antibody or protein specifically created by white blood cells after they come into contact with a foreign cell or other object. Antibodies fight infections and other dangerous foreign cells such as cancer cells by surrounding the cell so it is eventually expelled from the body or outright killing the abnormal material.

Special Populations

Teenagers

Smoking frequently begins in early adolescence. The first experimentation usually occurs prior to age 12. Eighty percent of all smokers started smoking before the age of 18. According to the Center for Disease Control and Prevention (CDC), the current estimates are that over 4000 teens between the ages of 12 and 17 become regular smokers every day. Half of these teens will become daily smokers. One out of 11 8th-graders smoke, and 1 out of 4 12th- graders smoke. There is no typical social pattern, although many of the teen smokers exhibit low self-esteem and problems adjusting socially.

Teens get addicted faster than adults. Some researchers believe that because the brains of adolescents are still developing, they can become more easily addicted. Only a few trials with cigarettes can hook a teenager, as little as a couple of cigarettes within a period of months. (Question 33 has additional information about how long it takes for someone to become addicted.) Some statistics about teens and smoking are:

- 33% of teenagers reported symptoms of addiction when smoking only one day a month
- 49% of teens reported addiction by the time they were smoking one day a week
- 70% of adolescents who are daily smokers stated that they are addicted

Factors that contribute to teen smoking are:

- Availability and access to tobacco products
- The perception that smoking is "cool"
- Parental smoking
- Peer smoking

Young Adults

Although tobacco use among teens is of great concern to adolescent advocates, parents, and teachers, the fact is that young adults are the group with the largest numbers of addicted smokers: 44.3% of those ages 18 to 25 use tobacco. This is the largest group of smokers for any age group. Many of these young people started to smoke when they were children or teens.

College Students

Although the prevalence of smoking has begun to decline starting in 2000, many students who started smoking as children or teens continue to do so. White students smoke more than other ethnic groups, and both male and female college students smoke at similar rates.

Elderly

Most seniors who continue to smoke became addicted to tobacco when they were young. Consequently, many have health problems related to smoking. Here are some facts. Smokers who are seniors are more prone to osteoporosis, which contributes to the 850,000 fractures among those over age 65 in the United States, of which 300,000 are hip fractures. Persons with hip fractures have a higher death rate by 12% to 20%.

Smoking is related to cataracts, which is the leading cause of blindness among the elderly worldwide and the leading cause of visual loss in the United States. Smokers have two to three times the risk of developing cataracts than nonsmokers.

The prevalence of chronic obstructive pulmonary disease (COPD) is consistently among the top 10 problems encountered by elderly smokers. The prevalence is highest in men and women over age 65.

89. What are the rates of smoking between socioeconomic groups and educational levels?

During the Depression era and afterwards, as the consumer culture emerged, cigarettes gained popular approval as a national product that crossed the boundaries of class, gender, race, and ethnicity. However, that attitude began to change as the educated public became aware of the *Surgeon General's Report* linking cigarette smoking with lung cancer and other diseases (see Question 21).

By 1986, smoking became increasingly associated with lower educational and socioeconomic status. Data from the Centers for Disease Control and Prevention (CDC) demonstrated that smoking declines with increasing levels of education. More than 40% of people who dropped out of high school are smokers compared to 15% of those with college degrees. A researcher from the University of Michigan believes that smoking-related diseases will increasingly become a class-based phenomenon. Today, the number of smokers remains high only among the poor and the poorly educated.

90. Are the mentally ill more at risk of addiction to nicotine?

There are no gender differences among the mentally ill in terms of the percentage of smokers. Smoking among mentally ill patients is disproportionately high compared to the general population. People who suffer from a mental illness smoke over 44% of the cigarettes purchased in the United States. They are twice as likely to smoke as those who are not mentally ill. A very high percentage of the mentally ill will die of a tobacco-related disease.

People who suffer from a mental illness smoke over 44% of the cigarettes purchased in the United States.

Smoking cigarettes may be a form of self-medication because nicotine has a powerful influence on mood and cognition. (Questions 83 and 91 have further details about nicotine's possible health benefits and impact on mental illness.) Tobacco products may be treating both the psychiatric symptoms and the side effects of the medications used to treat the psychiatric disorders. Antipsychotic medications, in particular, which are used to treat schizophrenia, deliberately target dopamine in the brain by blocking its receptors. This has the unfortunate effect of negatively impacting dopamine transmission throughout the brain, including those areas related to attention and cognition. Smoking, which boosts dopamine, may be a way for patients taking these medications to reverse some of those negative effects. This is why psychiatric units in hospitals were the last hospital units to prohibit smoking.

More patients with depression smoke as well, and there is some evidence that nicotine receptors may play an important role in depression. A small study in 2006 at Duke University found that nonsmokers suffering from depression had improvement in some of their depressive symptoms after administering a nicotine patch. Finally, it has been well known that patients with ADHD are prone to addiction when they reach adulthood. The most common addiction is nicotine, which (as discussed in Questions 10, 32, and 91) is a potent stimulant. Smoking improves attention in these patients as well as others suffering from similar cognitive problems.

PART SEVEN

Surviving

I don't like gaining weight when I stop smoking. Why do I gain weight? What can I do about it?

I have so many pleasant memories of smoking. How can I create unpleasant memories about it?

Why do I need to gain support from family, friends, and others to succeed?

More . . .

91. I don't like gaining weight when I stop smoking. Why do I gain weight? What can I do about it?

The short answer is nicotine is a stimulant and all stimulants play a role in appetite suppression and weight loss. The original diet pills were all amphetamine derivatives (stimulants) and were routinely prescribed in the 1950s and 1960s until it became clear they were addictive. Stimulants partly work by increasing the basal metabolic rate, so you burn calories at a faster rate. Thus, when you stop taking them your metabolic rate slows down and you gain weight. Most of the newer medications that are used as weight control pills are also modified derivatives of amphetamines. These include the drug **fenfluramine**, more commonly remembered as the partner drug known as Fen-Phen that was removed from the market because of heart valve problems. Meridia (the trade name for the drug, sibutramine), instead of causing a direct release of norepinephrine as do the traditional stimulants, blocks the reuptake of norepinephrine and serotonin. Sibutramine is similar in action to some other antidepressant medications, and for that reason it is strongly advised not to use this if you are already taking an antidepressant. There is no real substitute for a strong diet and exercise program, as medications have limited benefits and significant side effects.

The more complicated answer regarding nicotine and weight comes from nicotine's unique actions on various other neurotransmitter and hormonal systems that affect weight, some of which are discussed briefly in Question 83. An additional neurotransmitter system that researchers are working on to aid in weight control may be surprising. Researchers are investigating the use of combination agents, including nicotine replacement therapies and a drug that targets the cannabinoid system. It has long been known that marijuana causes an increase in appetite and weight. A new drug, rimonabant, which is a reverse agonist at one of the cannabinoid receptors (CB1), was approved for use in the European Union (EU) as

Fenfluramine

A chemical structurally related to amphetamine but it causes an increase in serotonin and decreases appetite. Fenfluramine was originally released in combination with another chemical as Fen-Phen, a diet pill that was taken off the market in 1997 out of concerns that it affected heart valves.

a weight loss pill. There is some evidence to support its use as a smoking cessation agent in addition to its anorectic effects, but the EU has yet to approve its use in this arena.

Its application to the FDA for use in the United States was withdrawn over concerns about possible adverse effects—most notably depression, suicidal thinking, and self injurious behavior—but also due to the concern that it could lead to neurodegenerative disorders such as multiple sclerosis and Huntington's disease. Still, the fact that a variety of systems are involved in nicotine's effects on appetite and weight point out that this seemingly simple chemical has a very complex and still not well understood effect on the body and brain.

Some diet experts recommend the use of diet patches in addition to a nicotine patch. The ingredients of a typical diet patch are as follows:

1. Fucus vesiculosus, believed to increase the body's metabolism through stimulation of the thyroid, burn more calories, and enhance digestion.

2. Guarana, a caffeine-like stimulant that also helps to increase the metabolism while keeping energy levels high.

3. 5-Hydroxytryptophan (5-HTP), which helps control sweet and carbohydrate cravings by controlling serotonin levels in the brain.

4. Zinc pyruvate, which assists in the breakdown of fat cells while helping to build lean muscle mass.

5. Dehydroepiandrosterone (DHEA), which helps the body to manage the intake of calories more efficiently.

6. Yerba mate, a caffeine-like stimulant with appetite suppressant properties from South America.

7. Lecithin, which helps to break down fats and cholesterol and balance body weight.

8. Flaxseed oil, which keeps a balance of essential fatty acids for healthier dieting.

9. L-Carnitine, which increases the body's fat burning capabilities.

10. Zinc citrate, an essential mineral often lost when losing weight.

Again, there is no real substitute for a solid diet and exercise program, as they will not only help with the weight gain but will also help with the psychological effects of nicotine withdrawal. If you increase your exercise, drink plenty of fluids, and eat a balanced and healthy diet, you should be able to keep your weight under control and feel better to boot!

Lisa's comment:

I learned quickly that I'd rather diet and exercise later than have a lung disease that I may never survive. My health professional made me aware early on of how serious smoking is compared to dealing with weight gain. Besides, exercising took my mind off smoking, and I could run for over an hour (on a machine) after quitting smoking as compared to running for 14 minutes in the past.

92. Are there any long-term psychological or emotional symptoms that I should expect long after I stop smoking?

While the experience of loss and having mild symptoms of the blues is common during the immediate period following stopping smoking even after the withdrawal symptoms have passed, regardless of whether one takes NRT (less so when one is treated with bupropion or nortriptyline, which are antidepressants), a few people slip into a depression. More serious symptoms of depression include sleep and appetite disturbance, and feelings of guilt, helplessness, and hopelessness. Most serious is the development of thoughts of suicide that may include developing a plan without carrying it out (which medically is termed suicidal ideation) or thoughts of self-injury. If you find that the depression continues for more than a couple of weeks, especially when accompanied by any of the listed symptoms, you should call your doctor.

But more often than not, the long-term emotional consequences are positive. This comes from the elated feeling of successfully conquering what can only be described as the Mount Everest of addictions.

93. What can I do to ease any residual psychological or emotional pain short of taking medication?

This is the primary reason individual and group therapy improves smoking cessation rates! You can take proactive measures to enhance your sense of well-being so the cravings are less severe. Regular aerobic exercise (such as swimming, dancing, running, walking, etc.) stimulates breathing faster, precipitates perspiration, increases the heart rate, and releases **endorphins** ("feel good chemicals" secreted by the hypothalamus in the brain and pituitary gland following exercise). Plan regular exercise and follow the plan. Research shows that smokers who take up a regular exercise program have a much higher quit-smoking success rate. The greater the level of physical activity the higher the success rate at remaining tobacco-free. Many people use cigarettes to alleviate stress. Exercise is an excellent stress reliever and can replace your dependence on cigarettes for stress relief.

Eat a well-balanced diet. Drink lots of fluids. Any kind of fluids are good except coffee and alcohol, which often are triggers for a craving to smoke. Get more rest. Go to bed earlier than your usual bedtime to cope with the fatigue. Take a multivitamin for an energy boost.

Talk to yourself about the benefits of not smoking. Dispute all of the rationalizations that you used to remain a smoker. Reframe your thinking. Tell yourself, "I didn't give up smoking, I choose to become a nonsmoker, and this has been the greatest accomplishment of my life!" Visualize how much better you will look and feel. Meditate. Sit in a comfortable chair. Close your eyes. Make your mind a blank, allow all thoughts

More often than not, the long-term emotional consequences are positive.

Surviving

Endorphins

(Also known as endogenous opiates.) A type of natural opiate manufactured by the body after strenuous exercise, laughing, or excitement to act on a variety of physiological changes, including pain perception, appetite suppression, and elevated mood.

and feelings to fade into the background. Breathe slowly and deeply. After a couple of minutes, the craving to smoke will go away. Reward yourself with doing activities you like to do. Reach out to others; helping them will help you. Stay away from places where you smoked. Change your daily routine. Avoid smoke-filled rooms and friends who smoke. Explain to them your plan. Develop an action plan. Who do I want to be and what do I want to do, now that I am no longer a "smoker?" What are my goals? **Table 14** may help you to think about and identify your personal strategies for success.

Table 14   Action Plan

Goals	Strategies Needed to Achieve the Goals
Career	
Educational	
Non-work related	
Financial	
Emotional	
Spiritual	
Family (interpersonal)	
Goals for the month	
Goals for the year	
Long-term goals	
Other	

94. I have so many pleasant memories of smoking. How can I create unpleasant memories about it?

A form of conscious reprogramming is needed to replace the automatic pleasant memories with unpleasant ones. This is part of how cognitive behavioral therapy (CBT) works, in replacing the automatic negative thoughts associated with one's depression with positive thoughts (see Questions 71–73). However, this is especially challenging because it is replacing automatic pleasant memories associated with one's smoking with negative ones. Here is a list of unpleasant memories that one can attempt to conjure up whenever confronted with a positive memory. Obviously the list is neither comprehensive nor specific to every individual. It is important to write down your own list and practice them by reading the list out loud in addition to recalling as vividly as possible the sights, sounds, and odors associated with them.

- Struggling to hide the odor to avoid discovery and chastisement.
- Smoke seeping into everything, leaving its telltale signs including the grungy yellow tinge wherever it touched.
- The extra time and energy it took to buy cigarettes and smoke them.
- Running out of cigarettes in the middle of the night, running to the store to buy some.
- Smoking butts that tasted terrible because you ran out of cigarettes.
- Coughing when you first get up in the morning and periodically throughout the day.
- Holes in your clothes.
- Stains on your fingers.
- Burns on the furniture.
- Foul-smelling breath.

- Complaints from family, friends, and colleagues.
- Reminding yourself that cigarettes actually taste bad.
- Reminding yourself that smoking makes your body toxic, shortens your life, and can kill you with a terrible disease.

Joseph's comment:

The good memories were so long ago that I have a hard time recalling them. I enjoyed having a cigarette with my coffee in the morning, and when I was younger, I loved fitting in with the smoking crowd of my friends. It was the "adult" thing to do! The bad memories; my health was declining with smoker's cough in the morning; the price of cigarettes, consuming more and more of my monthly income; it becoming less and less the "cool" thing to do; and personal experience of loved ones dying of smoking-related ailments.

Lisa's comment:

With the help of my smoking cessation leader, I calculated that I was easily spending $50 a week (back in 2002!). After quitting, I soon justified buying a new stove and a new refrigerator! I got new clothes and "toys." I've been nicer to me ever since.

95. What is the Master Settlement Agreement?

The Master Settlement Agreement (MSA) awarded billions of dollars to the states in November 1998. The largest four tobacco companies made a cash settlement and agreed to amend other corporate practices in response to lawsuits brought by the Attorney Generals of 46 U.S. states and 5 U.S. territories. These tobacco companies also agreed to finance anti-smoking campaigns. This agreement occurred over multiple lawsuits alleging that the tobacco companies had been deceitful in their advertising campaign claims that smoking was safe and non-addictive. These allegations included illegal marketing campaigns directed to children.

The MSA specifically bans:

- The use of cartoon characters in advertising, promoting, packaging, or labeling of cigarettes;
- Billboards, stadium signs, and transit signs advertising cigarettes;
- Brand-logoed apparel and other merchandise (such as caps and T-shirts);
- Free-product sampling anywhere except for a facility or enclosed area where the operator ensures or has a reasonable basis to believe that no minors are present;
- Payments for use of cigarettes in movies, TV programs, live recorded performances, videos, or video games;
- Use of non-tobacco brand names on cigarettes (unless such use predated July 1, 1998);
- Licensing of third parties to use or advertise any cigarette brand name in a manner that would constitute a violation of the MSA if done by the participating manufacturer;
- Agreements that prohibit a third party from selling, purchasing, or displaying advertising discouraging the use of cigarettes or exposure to secondhand smoke;
- The use of a cigarette brand name as part of the name of a stadium or arena.

The MSA limits tobacco sponsorships to one per year and prohibits:

- Brand-name sponsorship of events with a significant youth audience;
- Sponsorship of events where the paid participants or contestants are youth;
- Sponsorship of concerts (unless events are age-restricted);
- Sponsorship of athletic events between opposing teams in any football, baseball, soccer, or hockey league.

With respect to any brand-name sponsorship allowed by the MSA:

- Advertising of the brand-name sponsorship event cannot advertise any cigarette;
- No participating manufacturer may refer to a brand-name sponsorship event or to a celebrity or other person in such an event in its advertising of cigarettes.

The MSA requires that:

- Tobacco-industry documents be publicly available through a Web site paid for by the companies;
- Tobacco companies disclose payments to lobbyists and other major donations.

The MSA disbanded the Tobacco Institute, the Council for Tobacco Research, and the Council for Indoor Air Research, and provides for regulation and oversight of any new trade organizations. In addition, the MSA restricts participating manufacturers from:

- Supporting diversion of MSA proceeds to any program that is neither tobacco related nor health related;
- Opposing legislation prohibiting the sale of cigarettes in packages less than 20;
- Opposing the passage of certain kinds of state and local legislation relating primarily to youth access to tobacco.

Over a 25-year period, the states will be receiving approximately $246 billion from tobacco companies through the MSA and four other individual state settlements that can be used to support anti-smoking efforts. Future annual payments, based upon inflation and cigarette sales, will continue in perpetuity. The MSA provides industry funding specifically earmarked for anti-youth-smoking education programs and a national health research foundation. As part of the $246 billion MSA, the participating tobacco companies agreed to pay approximately $1.45 billion to the states over 5 years for the creation and execution of an anti-smoking advertising and public education campaign designed to reduce and prevent teen smoking; and make contributions of $250 million over 10 years to a research foundation, which will be dedicated to the study of programs to reduce youth smoking as well as the study of and educational programs to prevent tobacco-related illnesses. Compliance is enforced by each state's attorney general. Failure to comply with these rules and restrictions can result in broad, court-ordered injunctions and civil penalties.

96. What have been the results of the Master Settlement Agreement since the settlement occurred?

The purpose was to help the states recover Medicare and Medicaid costs for publicly insured victims of tobacco-related diseases. By signing the MSA, states' attorneys general gave up the right to make legal claims against the tobacco companies for violating state antitrust laws and laws related to consumer protections. The participating tobacco companies agreed to change their marketing strategies to avoid advertising directly or indirectly to minors. Over the years, the tobacco companies have continued to meet their obligations in two ways: (1) by reimbursing the states for healthcare costs incurred from tobacco use, and (2) by showing they have increased spending on youth anti-smoking programs in the amount of $100 million annually.

The settlement prompted the companies to raise the price of tobacco. Following the agreement, the four principal tobacco companies—Philip Morris, R.J. Reynolds, Brown & Williamson, and Lorillard—raised their prices more than 45¢ per pack to cover the additional costs. The higher costs lead to a reduction in teenage smoking. The rates of smoking among American adolescents have reached their lowest point in nearly three decades, following the increased cost of cigarettes plus the development of anti-smoking educational programs.

97. Am I eligible for any legal compensation for a smoking-related illness since the MSA?

The intent of the MSA was to shield tobacco companies from further liability. However there have continued to be a number of lawsuits filed since the MSA was established in 1998. Some of these lawsuits have been class action, where a group or class of individuals is represented by an attorney and any awards are distributed across the class, including those who may not have directly been involved in the litigation. Other lawsuits have been individual, with the award going entirely to the individual or his or her estate. Whether or not a particular lawsuit is class action or individual is largely determined by the state where the group or individual resides. In 2004, a New York jury awarded $20 million to the wife of a long-term smoker who died of lung cancer. This was the first time in the history of New York that such litigation occurred. The most recent case, *Philip Morris v. Williams*, was heard by the Supreme Court in 2006 with a decision rendered February 20, 2007. In that case, an Oregon jury had awarded the widow of a deceased smoker $79.5 million in punitive damages. The defendant, Philip Morris, argued successfully that this was tantamount to taking property without due process and the Supreme Court reversed the decision on the award.

A plethora of Web sites feature personal injury attorneys supporting your right to sue, including those who specialize in tobacco. These lawsuits vary from state to state as civil laws differ in each state. As recently as 2002, for example, in California one could sue tobacco companies for fraud and negligence. Evidence that the industry altered tobacco with additives to make it more addictive would be admissible regardless of the industries' past protection from lawsuits. Most of these lawsuits, particularly since the master settlement agreement, have been unsuccessful. The Supreme Court reversal is but one example. In 2005, the Illinois Supreme Court reversed a $10 billion judgment against a tobacco company regarding the misleading statements that light cigarettes were safer to use. In January 2008, the Florida Supreme Court mandated a filing deadline for all tobacco related injury cases, as it would no longer hear any cases submitted after that date. The bottom line is that the window of opportunity is running out and one must first consult an attorney before proceeding further.

98. Why do I need to gain support from family, friends, and others to succeed?

It is critical that you share your plan with your family and friends and to elicit their support in order to give you the best chance of success. Studies repeatedly demonstrate that supports improve success rates significantly compared to patients who quit without the use of supports. (Questions 60 and 73 have further information on the importance of supports.) It has been repeatedly demonstrated that the majority of our habitual behaviors are strongly reinforced or extinguished because of our social supports. Humans are social animals. This is why peer groups have such a powerful influence on youth. This is also the reason advertisers utilize celebrities to pitch their products. We want to be like them so we copy their preferences to feel more like them. Family, church, and community are discussed so much by politicians as reinforcing core values because of this fact. You will need the encouragement of others as you proceed with your plan to quit.

Besides obtaining the support of family and friends, you may also find a support group or a "buddy" to give you additional personal support. Make a date with your buddy either in person or by phone. If you develop a relationship with a buddy, phone each other daily, at least until you are over the initial period of withdrawal. Many hospitals have support groups or smoking cessation programs. You can call your local hospital, the American Lung Association, or the American Cancer Society, or look on the Internet for names and places where there are support groups and/or to find a telephone hotline.

Studies repeatedly demonstrate that supports improve success rates significantly compared to patients who quit without the use of supports.

99. In case I can't get in touch with my buddy or family members, is there a 24-hour hotline I can call?

Yes there is! In November of 2004, The National Cancer Institute Information Service (NCI/CIS) developed a network of telephone assistance hotlines in order to counsel smokers who wish to quit smoking. Through this network, states received funding as part of the Center for Disease Control's Tobacco Control Program so that there was money to establish hotlines known as quitlines or to expand existing telephone assistance counseling programs. **The National Quit Line telephone number is 1-800-Quit Now OR 1-800-784-8669**, which will transfer you to your own local geographical area. Additionally, many local smoking cessation programs offer hotlines 24/7. Look online or in the Yellow Pages of your phone book, or call your local hospital to find out where and whom to call for information about a hotline number.

100. Where can I find more information?

The following list of resources and organizations have more information about quitting smoking.

The National Cancer Institute (NCI)
1-800 4-CANCER (422-6230)

The American Cancer Society (ACS)
http://www.cancer.org

The American Heart Association
1-800-AHA-USA1 (1-800-242-8721)
http://www.americanheart.org/

The American Lung Association
1-800-LUNG-USA (1-800-586-4872)
http://www.lungusa.org/
http://www.lungassoc.org/

The National Institute on Drug Abuse (NIDA)
http://www.nida.nih.gov/

The Department of Public Health (DOPH) and the American Public Health Association (APHA)
202-777-APHA (1-202-777-2742)

The Agency for Health Care Policy and Research (AHCPR)
U.S. Department of Health and Human Services (DHHS)
1-800-358-9295
http://www.ahcpr.gov/

The American Council on Science and Health (ACSH)
http://www.acsh.org/

Bureau of Alcohol, Tobacco, Firearms and Explosives (BATF)
1-202-927-8210
http://www.atf.treas.gov/

Centers for Disease Control and Prevention (CDC)
National Center of Chronic Disease Prevention and Health Promotion (NCCDPHP), Office of Smoking and Health (OSH)
1-770-488-5701 (general information/publication requests)
1-800-CDC-1311 (media campaign response line/fax service).
http://www.cdc.gov/tobacco/

Doctors Ought to Care (DOC)
http://www.fammed.wisc.edu/med-student/doc

The Federal Trade Commission (FTC)
1-202-326-2222 (publications)
1-202-326-3090 (tobacco-related questions)
http://www.ftc.gov/

Food and Drug Administration (FDA)
1-301-827-4420
http://www.fda.gov/

Surviving

The National Health Information Center (NHIC)
1-800-336-4797
1-301-565-4167
http://www.health.gov/nhic

The Agency for Health Care Policy and Research (AHRQ)
1-800-358-9295
http://www.surgeongeneral.gov/tobacco/

The American Society of Addiction Medicine (ASAM)
1-301-656-3920
http://www.asam.org/

Web Site Information

Mayo Clinic Nicotine Dependence Center
http://www.mayoclinic.org/ndc-rst/

Tobacco.org
Tobacco news and information: http://www.tobacco.org/
Tobacco control groups: http://www.tobacco.org/Resources/
tob_adds.html

Tobacco Control Archives from the University of California,
San Francisco (UCSF)
http://www.library.ucsf.edu/tobacco/tcafaq.html

Action on Smoking and Health (ASH)
http://www.ash.org/
List of state tobacco control organizations: http://www.ash
.org/websites.html

truth
http://www.thetruth.com

Nicotine Anonymous (a 12-step self-help group)
1-800-415-0328
http://www.nicotine-anonymous.org

QuitNet, quit all together
http://www.quitnet.org

Seventh Day Adventist's support groups

Smokers Anonymous (available through Alcoholics Anonymous)

SmokEnders
http://www.smokenders.com

Learn how to Quit Smoking, Get Expert Help, Access Print Resources, Find Studies
http://www.smokefree.gov/

Smoking Cessation Leadership Center
http://smokingcessationleadership.ucsf.edu/

National Mental Health Information Center, Substance Abuse and Mental Health
http://mentalhealth.samhsa.gov/

The Foundation for a Smoke Free America
http://www.anti-smoking.org/

The National Clearinghouse for Drug and Alcohol Information (NCDAI)
http://ncadi.samhsa.gov/

Public Citizen, Tobacco News Resources
http://www.citizen.org (and enter tobacco in search engine)

Centers for Disease Control and Prevention, Smoking and Tobacco Use
http://www.cdc.gov/tobacco

Quit For Life
http://www.freeclear.com/quit-for-life/

WebMD
http://www.webmd.com

WhyQuit.com
http://www.whyquit.com/

Philip Morris USA, QuitAssist™ Program
http://www2.philipmorrisusa.com/en/quitassist/index_flash
.asp

Corporate Accountability International
http://www.stopcorporateabuse.org/cms/

Appendix

TABLE 15 Recommended Medications for Smoking Cessation and Their Success Rates

Non-NRT Medication	Success Rates	NRT Medication	Success Rates
Bupropion XL (Wellbutrin) 150 mg–300 mg/d	24.2%	Nicotine Gum	26.1%
Varenicline (Chantix) 1 mg/d	25.4%	Nicotine Patch	23.7%
2 mg/d	33.2%	Nicotine Nasal Spray	26.7%
Nortriptyline 50 mg–150 mg/d	22.5%	Nicotine Inhaler	24.8%
Clonidine 0.1–0.3 mg/d	25.0%	Nicotine Lozenge 2 mg/d 4 mg/d	24.2% 23.6%
Placebo	13.8%		

References

How We Get Addicted; Lemonick, Michael D.; *Time*, July 5, 2007. http://www.time.com/time/printout/0,8816,1640436,00.html.

Hooked From The First Cigarette; DeFranza, Joseph; *Scientific American*, May 2008, pp 82-87.

Nicotine as Therapy; Powledge, Tabitha M; *PLoS Biol*, November 2004; 2(11): e404. Published online 2004, November 16. doi: 10.1371/journal.pbio.0020404

Glossary

A

Acetylcholine: A neurotransmitter found in both the peripheral nervous system (PNS) and the central nervous system (CNS). In the PNS, it is involved in both muscle contraction as well as that part of the involuntary nervous system involved with "rest and restoration." In the CNS, it is involved with memory function.

Acetylcholine Receptor Subtypes: The two major subtypes include muscarinic and nicotinic, but each has its own multiple subtypes. These are located throughout the nervous system and each subtype is specific for a different type of drug as well as acetylcholine.

Acetylcholinesterase: An enzyme that breaks down acetylcholine, rendering it inactive. Blocking this enzyme leads to a relative increase in acetylcholine.

Acrolein: Responsible for the gummy yellowish residue and acrid smell from burning cigarettes. It is considered carcinogenic and is toxic to the skin. It was used in chemical warfare during World War I.

Adrenal Medulla: The central part of the adrenal gland surrounded by the adrenal cortex. It produces adrenalin (also known as epinephrine), norepinephrine, and dopamine. It responds to stress and is part of the sympathetic, "fight or flight" nervous system.

Adrenergic Receptors: Also known as adrenoreceptors. Alpha- and beta-adrenergic adrenoreceptors are the subtypes of adrenergic receptors responsible for various physiological responses at their site of action. They are part of the sympathetic nervous system.

Alkaloids: Naturally occurring chemical compounds containing basic nitrogen atoms that are produced by a large variety of organisms, including bacteria, fungi, plants, and animals.

Alpha-Bungarotoxin: A snake venom that binds irreversibly to nicotinic acetylcholine receptors at the neuromuscular junction, causing paralysis and death.

Analgesia: A type of drug that relieves pain. Analgesics include nonsteroidal anti-inflammatory (NSAIDs) agents such as aspirin and opiates such as morphine.

Angina Pectoris: (Also known as angina.) Severe chest pain due to a blockage of blood flow in the arteries of the heart. It is a symptom of an impending heart attack.

Anticholinergic: A substance that blocks the effects of acetylcholine in the nervous system. Many of these drugs have side effects, including blurred vision, dry mouth, urinary hesitance, and constipation. It can also cause short-term memory problems.

Arrhythmias: Abnormal heart rhythms.

Atropine: (Also known as the deadly nightshade.) A substance from the plant *Atropa belladonna*, it blocks muscarinic acetylcholine receptors causing anticholinergic side effects. By blocking these receptors, essentially the parasympathetic action is decreased, leading to a relative increase in sympathetic action.

Attention Deficit Hyperactivity Disorder (ADHD): A persistent pattern of inattention and/or hyperactivity, impulsivity that is seen more frequently in children with ADHD than in children at comparable developmental levels. Other features associated with ADHD are low frustration tolerance, temper outbursts, stubbornness, excessive and frequent insistence on their own requests, labile mood swings, dysphoria, rejection by peers, and poor self-esteem. Academic achievement is often impaired due to being distractible. Conflicts with authority figures (both parents and school personnel) are common. Many of these children also have oppositional defiant disorders. These children may have been exposed to drugs or alcohol in utero. Many ADHD children exhibited low birth weights as newborns. Some teenagers who have ADHD self-medicate with drugs or alcohol.

Axon: That part of the neuron or nerve cell that is a long tube conducting neural signals away from the cell body.

B

Barbiturates: A class of drugs that affect GABA to prevent seizures from occurring. Used for anxiety disorder until the discovery of benzodiazepines, which were found to be much safer in overdose.

Benzodiazepines: A class of anti-anxiety medications that include the drugs commonly known as Valium and Xanax.

Benzopyrene: A polycyclic aromatic hydrocarbon that is highly carcinogenic and found in tobacco tar. It is also found in charbroiled food and burnt toast.

Bidis: (Also known as Beedis.) A flavored cigarette common to India but exported worldwide. It is especially popular among U.S. teenagers.

Bronchodilator: A drug or chemical that relaxes the smooth muscle of the bronchi and bronchioles to open the airways, allowing more air to reach the lungs. Commonly prescribed in patients with airway diseases such as asthma and COPD.

Bronchus: The large airway of the lungs. No gas exchange between the lungs and the bloodstream occurs here.

Bupropion: Generic name for the drugs Wellbutrin, marketed as an antidepressant, and Zyban, marketed as a smoking cessation medication.

C

Cannabinoids: A group of compounds found in *Cannabis*, the marijuana plant, which are responsible for its psychoactive effects.

Carbon Monoxide: A tasteless, odorless, and colorless gas that binds tightly to hemoglobin in a manner similar to oxygen, thereby preventing oxygen from being transported to the organs. Intake of excess carbon monoxide leads to death. It is found in automobile emissions and cigarette smoke.

Catecholamines: Chemicals used as neurotransmitters and produced from the amino acid tyrosine. They include epinephrine, norepinephrine, and dopamine, all of which are produced in the brain as well as in the adrenal medulla, which is part of the sympathetic nervous system.

Chronic Bronchitis: Chronic inflammation of the bronchi that can be caused by an infection but more commonly is the result of COPD and chronic smoking.

Clonidine: A medication commonly prescribed for high blood pressure. It acts on the alpha-2 adrenoreceptors, which regulate the release of norepinephrine in the sympathetic nervous system. By stimulating these receptors, clonidine turns down the amount of epinephrine released and thus lowers blood pressure.

Cognitive Behavioral Therapy (CBT): A type of therapeutic intervention that reinforces "positive thinking" and extinguishes "negative thinking" to change undesirable thought patterns and eventually behaviors. Originally developed to treat depression to change faulty beliefs that cause errors in self-judgment and judgments about life. This therapeutic intervention has been found useful in the treatment of alcoholism and smoking cessation.

Colostrum: The first milk produced late in pregnancy and within the first few days of the baby's birth. It is also known as *immune milk* as it contains the mother's immunoglobulins, which are proteins from the mother's immune system that aid the infant to fight infection.

Contraindication: A condition or factor that increases the risk of an adverse event when taking a particular medication or receiving a particular treatment. A relative contraindication means that there are possibilities of receiving the medication/treatment without ill effects. An absolute contraindication means that such medication/treatment can never be received.

COPD (Chronic Obstructive Pulmonary Disease): (Also known as chronic airway disease.) A chronic lung condition brought on from cigarette smoking. It leads to a decrease in the lung's ability to oxygenate the body and often is progressive and irreversible.

Cortex: The outer membrane of an organ, such as the cerebral cortex of the brain or the adrenal cortex of the adrenal gland. It is used to identify a different part of an organ, which serves a different function for that organ.

Craving-Generation System: A hypothesized, yet to be proven part of the brain, the function of which is to generate craving for a particular object, such as food or drugs, which are addictive.

Craving-Inhibition System: A hypothesized, yet to be proven part of the brain, the function of which is to inhibit or turn off craving for a particular object, such as food or drugs, which are addictive.

Cytisine: A chemical produced from a variety of plants that has a mechanism of action similar to nicotine. It has been used on occasion in Eastern Europe as a smoking cessation agent. Varenicline is a synthetic analogue of cytisine.

Cytochrome P450 Enzymes: A group of enzymes found in the liver that function to break down chemicals for elimination from the body. These chemicals include but are not limited to medications. Some medications can block these enzymes while other medications or drugs, such as nicotine, can induce or accelerate these enzymes.

D

DMXB-A: A drug that activates the alpha-7 subtype of the nicotine receptor and is being used experimentally to improve cognition in patients with Alzheimer's disease and schizophrenia.

DNA (Deoxyribonucleic Acid): A type of nucleic acid molecule that contains a code of genetic instructions for the development and functioning in all living organisms and some viruses.

Dopamine: One of the brain's major neurotransmitters, dopamine is responsible for attention, alertness, decision making, reward, pleasure, and elevated mood.

Drug: A compound that, when ingested, alters bodily function in some manner.

Dysphoria: An unpleasant or uncomfortable mood, not necessarily depression, although it could be. It is the opposite of euphoria, a particularly good mood.

E

Electrochemical: The means by which the nerve conducts signals through the body. Chemical changes lead to electrical changes and vice versa.

Emphysema: A form of COPD where the lung tissue has lost elasticity. This causes the small airways to collapse decreasing the lung's ability to oxygenate the body.

Endorphins: (Also known as endogenous opiates.) A type of natural opiate manufactured by the body after strenuous exercise, laughing, or excitement to act on a variety of physiological changes, including pain perception, appetite suppression, and elevated mood.

Enzyme: A biological molecule that catalyzes or accelerates a chemical reaction. Most enzymes are proteins.

Epibatidine: A chemical produced by an Ecuadorian frog, found on its skin, which is 200 times more potent as an analgesic than morphine but acts on nicotinic acetylcholine receptors.

Epinephrine: (Also known as the hormone adrenaline.) A catecholamine derived from tyrosine, an amino acid, which is produced in the adrenal medulla and released into the bloodstream to activate the "fight or flight" response via the sympathetic nervous system.

Euphoria: An emotion that is a state of intense happiness and feelings of well-being.

F

FDA (Food and Drug Administration): The Federal Agency devoted to ensuring the safety and effectiveness of all medications released in the United States.

Fenfluramine: A chemical structurally related to amphetamine, but it causes an increase in serotonin and decreases appetite. Fenfluramine was originally released in combination with another chemical as Fen-Phen, a diet pill that was taken off the market in 1997 out of concerns that it affected heart valves.

FEV1 (Forced Expiratory Volume in One Second): Part of a set of measures collectively called pulmonary function tests that allow physicians to measure lung function. FEV1 measures the total volume of air exhaled in one second.

fMRI (Functional Magnetic Resonance Imaging): A type of noninvasive imaging study that allows the observer to visualize the areas of the brain that are functioning after exposure to a particular brain activity.

G

GABA (Gamma Amino Butyric Acid): The brain's major inhibitory neurotransmitter. This neurotransmitter dampens all brain activity, essentially calming the brain down at every level.

Ganglion: A mass of tissue, generally nervous, which provides relay points and intermediary connections between different neurological structures in the body, such as the peripheral and central nervous systems.

Ginseng: Literally, "man-root" in Chinese for its distinctive form resembling the legs of a human. It is used in traditional Chinese medicine as a muscle relaxant and stimulant.

Glutamate: The brain's major excitatory neurotransmitter. This neurotransmitter activates all brain activity, essentially stimulating the brain and "lifting" it up at every level.

Glycogen: A series of glucose (or sugar) molecules attached together in what is known as a polysaccharide. It is produced and stored in the liver and utilized by the body during times when short bursts of energy are required, such as in the "fight or flight" response.

Gray Matter: The part of the brain that contains the nerve cell bodies, including the cell nucleus and its metabolic machinery, as opposed to the *axons*, which are essentially the "transmission wires" of the nerve cell. The cerebral cortex contains the gray matter.

H

Homeostasis: A property of most living systems, which are organized to maintain a stable, balanced state of equilibrium.

Hookah: A water pipe used for smoking tobacco, found principally in Middle Eastern cultures.

Hormone: A chemical produced by the body and released into the bloodstream that has metabolic effects on cells at other sites in the body.

Huntington Disease: An inherited (genetic) disorder affecting the nervous system. It leads to a degeneration of nerves that impact both the motor system and mental functioning. Characteristics are abnormal involuntary motor movements, dementia, and eventually death. It is a neurodegenerative disorder.

Hypercoagulability: A tendency for blood to clot too easily, which can lead to stroke or other types of vascular disease.

Hypothalamus: Located below the thalamus, just above the brain stem, this part of the brain links the nervous system to the endocrine system via the pituitary gland. It is responsible for certain metabolic processes and other activities of the autonomic nervous system, particularly the sympathetic "fight or flight" response.

I

Immunoglobulin: An antibody or protein specifically created by white blood cells after they come into contact with a foreign cell or other object. Antibodies fight infections and other dangerous foreign cells such as cancer cells by surrounding the cell so it is eventually expelled from the body or outright killing the abnormal material.

K

Kava: The extract from a plant found primarily in the Pacific Islands. It is marketed as an herbal medicine against stress, insomnia, and anxiety.

L

Limbic Area: A set of brain structures that includes the hippocampus, amygdala, and anterior thalamic nuclei that support a variety of functions including emotion, behavior, and long-term memory. These structures are closely associated with the olfactory structures.

Lipolysis: The breakdown of fat stored in fat cells.

Lobelia: (Also known as asthma weed or pukeweed.) A plant substance used by Native Americans medicinally to treat respiratory and muscle disorders, and as a purgative. Today it is used to treat asthma and food poisoning, and is often used as part of smoking cessation programs. It is a physical relaxant, and can serve as a nerve depressant, easing tension and panic.

M

Motivational Interviewing (MI): A brief treatment approach designed to produce rapid internally-motivated change in addictive behavior and other problem behaviors. The core principles are (a) to express empathy, (b) develop discrepancy, (c) avoid augmentation, (d) roll with resistance, and (e) support self-efficacy. MI assumes that ambivalence and fluctuating motivation occur during substance abuse recovery.

Multiple Sclerosis: A neurodegenerative disorder that affects the motor system and leads to weakness, paralysis, and death.

Muscarinic: Referring to muscarine, a chemical that stimulates acetylcholine receptors, located in the brain and the parasympathetic nervous system.

N

Naltrexone: Generic drug for ReVia. It is an opioid antagonist that competes with narcotics at opiate receptor sites, blocking the opioid analgesics. It is used as an antidote when there is respiratory distress induced by opiate intoxication and to treat opiate addiction.

Nerve (see neuron).

Neuromodulator: A process in which one neuron uses different neurotransmitters to connect to several neurons, as opposed to direct synaptic transmission where one neuron directly reaches another neuron. These transmitters are secreted by a small group of neurons and diffuse through large areas of the nervous system, affecting multiple neurons. Examples of neuromodulators include dopamine, serotonin, acetylcholine, histamine, and others.

Neuromuscular Junction: The junction of the axon terminal of a motor neuron with the muscle fiber responsible for ultimately causing the muscle to contract. In vertebrates, the signal passes through the neuromuscular junction via the neurotransmitter acetylcholine and is a nicotinic receptor.

Neuron: A nerve cell made up of a cell body with extensions called dendrites and the axon.

Neuroplasticity: Changes that occur in the organization of the brain as a result of experience.

Neurotransmitters: Chemicals released by nerves that communicate with other nerves causing electrochemical changes in those nerves to continue to propagate a signal.

Nicotiana rustica: One of the principal nicotine-containing plants that has been cultivated as a source of tobacco. Although it has a higher nicotine content and is harsher, it is used principally for the insecticide industry.

Nicotiana tabacum: The tobacco plant.

Nicotine: A chemical found in a variety of plants that targets a specific group of acetylcholine receptors known as nicotinic receptors.

Nicotinic receptors: Short for nicotinic acetylcholine receptors, they form ion-gated channels in certain neurons. They are located at the neuromuscular junction as well as on the postganglionic sympathetic and parasympathetic nervous system in the body. Stimulation of these receptors causes muscle contraction.

Nitrosamines: Nitrosamines are found in many foods, including beer, fish, and also in meat and cheese products preserved with nitrite pickling salt. They are also produced from grilling and frying food as well as from burning tobacco. Carcinogenic in a wide variety of animal species, a feature suggesting that they may also be cancer-causing in humans.

Norepinephrine: (Also known as noradrenaline.) A neurotransmitter located in the brain as well as a stress hormone released by the adrenal glands. As a stress hormone, also known as epinephrine or adrenaline, this compound affects the "fight or flight" response by activating that part of the involuntary nervous system known as the sympathetic nervous system to increase heart rate, release energy from fat, and increase muscle readiness. As a neurotransmitter, it increases alertness and helps in elevating mood; it also can increase anxiety.

Nortriptyline: Generic drug for Pamelor, a tricyclic antidepressant medication that is recommended as a second-line non-NRT medication for smoking cessation.

NRT (Nicotine Replacement Therapy): Any type of aid to supplant the nicotine in tobacco use in an effort to wean from nicotine and stop the addiction.

Nuclei: Pleural for nucleus. A membrane-enclosed organelle that contains most of the cell's genetic material in DNA. The function of the nucleus is to maintain the integrity of genetic material and to control the activities of the cell by regulating genetic expression.

O

Opiate: A type of opioid. An opioid is any agent that binds to opioid receptors, found principally in the central nervous system and gastrointestinal tract. There are four broad classes of opioids: (1) endogenous opioid peptides, produced in the body; (2) opium alkaloids that are plant products, such as morphine (the prototypical opioid) and codeine; (3) semi-synthetic opioids such as heroin and oxycodone; and (4) fully synthetic opioids such as methadone that have structures unrelated to the opium alkaloids. Although the term opiate is often used as a synonym for opioid, it is more properly limited to the natural opium alkaloids and the semi-synthetics derived from them.

P

Parasympathetic: The part of the peripheral nervous system called the autonomic or involuntary nervous system that controls the body's "rest and restoration" response. (Opposite to the sympathetic nervous system, which controls the body's "fight or flight" response.)

Partial Agonist: A chemical (such as a drug) that can both block and stimulate a receptor depending upon the relative amount of neurotransmitter present in the synaptic cleft. If the amount of neurotransmitter is large, the chemical acts as an antagonist, and if the amount of neurotransmitter is low, the chemical acts as an agonist.

Pathophysiology: The study of physiology focusing on disease processes.

Platelets: (Also known as thrombocytes.) A type of blood cell involved in the cellular mechanisms of the formation of blood clots. Low levels or dysfunction predisposes for bleeding, while high levels, although usually asymptomatic, may increase the risk of the development of a thrombus.

Polynuclear Aromatic Hydrocarbons: Chemicals found in oil, coal, and tar deposits, and are produced as byproducts of fuel burning (whether fossil fuel or biomass), including tobacco. Some of these compounds have been identified as carcinogenic.

Postganglionic: The beginning of the autonomic nervous system, which transmits from the central nervous system to the various organs. Nicotinic receptors are located here.

Preganglionic: The end of the central nervous system as it is communicating with the autonomic nervous system, which is part of the peripheral nervous system.

Psychoactive: A drug or chemical substance that acts on the brain to alter mood, behavior, perception, or consciousness. Abuse of some of these substances may cause addiction.

Psychosis: A state in which an individual experiences hallucinations, delusions, and disorganized thoughts, speech, and/or behaviors.

R

Radioactive Carcinogens: Those elements produced by tobacco smoke that are radioactive and therefore carcinogenic.

Receptor: Specific areas of protein on a neuron that are configured to respond only to specific neurotransmitters. Receptors act like locks that only can be opened by specific keys (the neurotransmitters).

Renin: A circulating enzyme that participates in regulating the body's blood pressure.

Reuptake: A transporter protein located presynaptically that serves to transport a neurotransmitter back up into the neuron, essentially ending transmission between two nerves.

Reynaud Syndrome: The result of vascular spasms that decrease blood supply to the respective regions. Smoking worsens the frequency and intensity of attacks, and there is a hormonal component.

Rimonabant: An anti-obesity drug that is an inverse agonist for the cannabinoid receptor CB1. Its main avenue of effect is reduction in appetite. The drug is available only in Europe. There is some suggestion that it may be useful in tobacco cessation and prevention of weight gain associated with smoking.

S

Schizophrenia: A psychiatric disorder that has symptoms of hallucinations and delusions associated with significant cognitive deficits, particularly in the area of social cognition but also in areas of the brain involving attention, concentration, and planning.

Sensitization-Homeostasis Theory: A theory of addiction involving two complementary systems, the craving-generation system and the craving-inhibition system, which helps to explain how a person can become addicted to tobacco after only a few cigarettes.

Serotonin: One of the brain's major neurotransmitters. Responsible for "vegetative functions" that include sleep, appetite, sex drive (libido), anxiety, and mood.

Sibutramine: (Also known as Meridia). A medication for the treatment of obesity that acts as an appetite suppressant. It is a centrally acting serotonin-norepinephrine reuptake inhibitor

structurally related to amphetamines but is not considered to be addictive.

SIDS (Sudden Infant Death Syndrome): (Also known as crib death or cot death.) The leading cause of unexplained death in apparently healthy infants aged one month to one year.

Synapse: The gap between nerves where neurotransmitters are released that allow nerves to communicate with one another.

T

Tar: That part of tobacco associated with a variety of toxic substances, notably nitrosamines, radioactive elements, acrolein, and polynuclear aromatic hydrocarbons.

TNCO (Tar, Nicotine, and Carbon Monoxide) Ceilings: The total upper value of the aerosol residue, nicotine, and carbon monoxide contents as measured by a cigarette smoking machine calibrated to ISO standards. This measure is used by countries worldwide to regulate manufactured tobacco products.

Trachea: The main airway from the mouth to the bronchi.

Transport Pump: A protein involved in reuptake of neurotransmitters.

Transtheoretical Model: A theoretical model of behavior change. The model involves emotions, cognitions, and behavior, and has several stages of change associated with it, including precontemplation, contemplation, preparation, action, and maintenance.

U

Up-Regulation: The process by which a cell increases the number of receptors to a given hormone or neurotransmitter to improve its sensitivity to this molecule. (A decrease of receptors is called down-regulation.)

V

Varenicline: Generic name for Chantix, a medication for smoking cessation. It is a partial nicotine agonist, acting to both stimulate the nicotine receptor as well as block the effects of additional nicotine. Thus, it serves a dual role in treating nicotine withdrawal as well as decreasing the pleasure one would derive from smoking while taking the medication.

W

White Matter: Nerve tissue in the brain and spinal chord that consists of axons and the sheaths (called myelin) covering the axons to carry nerve impulses between neurons within the nervous system.

Index